PARTNERSHIPS IN
FAMILY-CENTERED CARE

◆ ◆ ◆

PARTNERSHIPS IN FAMILY-CENTERED CARE
A Guide to
Collaborative Early Intervention ◆◆◆

by

PEGGY ROSIN, M.S., CCC-Sp.
University of Wisconsin–
Madison

AMY D. WHITEHEAD, B.S.
University of Wisconsin–
Madison

LINDA I. TUCHMAN, M.S.
University of Wisconsin–
Madison

GEORGE S. JESIEN, PH.D.
University of Wisconsin–
Madison

AUDREY L. BEGUN, PH.D.
University of Wisconsin–
Milwaukee

LIZ IRWIN, M.S.W.
Milwaukee Women's
Center, Inc.

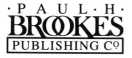

·P A U L·H·
BROOKES
PUBLISHING Cº

Baltimore • London • Toronto • Sydney

Paul H. Brookes Publishing Co., Inc.
Post Office Box 10624
Baltimore, Maryland 21285-0624

Typeset by Brushwood Graphics, Inc., Baltimore, Maryland.
Manufactured in the United States of America by
The Maple Press Co., York, Pennsylvania.

Permission to adapt the following is gratefully acknowledged:

Pages 22–23: List from Home-based early childhood services: Cultural sensitivity in a family systems approach by K. Wayman, E.W. Lynch, and M. Hanson (1990). *Topics in Early Childhood Special Education, 10*(4), 56–75. Copyright © 1990 by PRO-ED, Inc. Adapted and reprinted by permission.

The case studies described in this book are completely fictional. Any similarity to actual individuals or circumstances is coincidental and no implications should be inferred.

The photographs appearing in this volume were taken by Glenn Trudel. The photograph on the cover was taken by Amy D. Whitehead.

Library of Congress Cataloging-in-Publication Data
Partnerships in family-centered care : a guide to collaborative early
  intervention / by Peggy Rosin . . . [et al.].
      p.   cm.
  Includes bibliographical references and index.
  ISBN 1-55766-225-8
  1. Home-based family services—United States. I. Rosin, Peggy.
HV699.P324   1995
362.82'8'0973—dc20   95-31954
                                                                        CIP

British Library Cataloguing-in-Publication data are available from the British Library.

CONTENTS ◆◆◆

ABOUT THE AUTHORS ◆◆◆

Peggy Rosin, M.S., CCC-Sp., Project Coordinator, Pathways Service Coordination Project, Waisman Center, Room 619, University of Wisconsin–Madison, 1500 Highland Avenue, Madison, Wisconsin 53705-2280

Peggy Rosin is a distinguished outreach specialist at the Waisman Center Early Intervention Program at the University of Wisconsin–Madison. She has a wealth of experience in direct service, personnel preparation, and project management. Ms. Rosin coordinates two Early Education Programs for Children with Disabilities grants, which are focused on early intervention service coordination. She has a strong commitment to working in partnership with parents and has co-facilitated a series of Parent Project activities. Ms. Rosin is a speech-language pathologist who has worked for 2 decades with young children with disabilities in a variety of interdisciplinary settings. Her research interests and current writing have focused on speech intelligibility in people with Down syndrome.

Amy D. Whitehead, B.S., Project Coordinator, Family-Centered Interdisciplinary Training Project in Early Intervention, Waisman Center, Room 227, University of Wisconsin–Madison, 1500 Highland Avenue, Madison, Wisconsin 53705-2280

Amy D. Whitehead coordinates two interdisciplinary preservice grants for the Waisman Center Early Intervention Program at the University of Wisconsin–Madison. Ms. Whitehead's background and training are primarily founded on her experience as a parent of three children, the oldest of whom has a physical disability. She is active in planning, implementation, and evaluation of statewide early intervention personnel development. Ms. Whitehead has given national presentations, participated in team teaching university classes, facilitated workshops, and co-coordinated a series of skill-building opportunities for parents. She is particularly interested in parent involvement in early intervention, faculty–parent co-instruction, and service coordination.

Linda I. Tuchman, M.S., Coordinator, Wisconsin Personnel Development Project, Waisman Center, Room 275, University of Wisconsin–Madison, 1500 Highland Avenue, Madison, Wisconsin 53705-2280.

Linda I. Tuchman has worked in a variety of capacities with children with disabilities and their families since 1972. She is a special educator with service experience as a classroom teacher, service coordinator, and clinical consultant. She is employed at the Waisman Center of the University of Wisconsin–Madison, where she coordinates Wisconsin's Birth to Three Personnel Development Project and works with the Pathways: Service Coordination Inservice Project (a federally funded, U.S. Department of Education, early education in-service project). Ms. Tuchman focuses on early intervention training, technical assistance, and materials development. Some of her special interests include home-based services; inclusive child care; service coordination; supporting family involvement in early intervention, screening, evaluation, and assessment; play-based and activity-based intervention; team development; and personnel preparation. Ms. Tuchman is also a doctoral candidate in early childhood special education at the University of Wisconsin–Madison.

George S. Jesien, Ph.D., Director, Early Intervention Program, Waisman Center, University Affiliated Program, Room 225, University of Wisconsin–Madison, 1500 Highland Avenue, Madison, Wisconsin 53705-2280

George S. Jesien has been involved in early intervention for more than 20 years. He has worked in various capacities, including school psychologist, home visitor, project manager, and director of state and federally funded programs working on behalf of young children with special needs and their families. He directs the Early Intervention Program at the Waisman Center, a University Affiliated Program. The Early Intervention Program coordinates a series of federal, state, and locally funded projects focusing on personnel development, technical assistance, and resource development in support of family-centered services for young children with special needs and their families.

In 1994–1995, Dr. Jesien served as a Joseph P. Kennedy, Jr., Foundation Public Policy Fellow, working with the Senate Subcommittee on Disability Policy to assist in the reauthorization of the Individuals with Disabilities Education Act (IDEA). He also has had extensive international experience in early intervention program development and personnel preparation and has served as state and national president for the International Division for Early Childhood (DEC).

Audrey L. Begun, Ph. D., Associate Professor, School of Social Welfare, University of Wisconsin–Milwaukee, Post Office Box 786, Milwaukee, Wisconsin 53201

Audrey L. Begun received her doctoral degree in 1987 from the University of Michigan in social work and psychology. Dr. Begun also holds a master of social work degree in the area of families, children, and youth. She is an associate professor in the social work programs at the University of Wisconsin–Milwaukee. She has taught courses on family development, developmental disabilities, family policy, and human development. Dr. Begun has authored and co-authored several articles and book chapters about sibling relationships and siblings with a family member who has a developmental disability; the vulnerability, risk, and resilience model; the relationship of human development and prevention models; and adolescent substance abuse prevention. Dr. Begun is a co-principal investigator on two projects, one designed to evaluate approaches to prevention of violence against women and one that evaluates family-centered adolescent substance abuse prevention intervention.

Liz Irwin, M.S.W., Director, Birth to Three Program, Milwaukee Women's Center, 611 North Broadway, Milwaukee, Wisconsin 53202

Liz Irwin, who edited an earlier version of this book, currently directs the home-based Birth to Three Program at the Milwaukee Women's Center, Inc. Ms. Irwin ran a statewide training and advocacy program for parents of children with disabilities for 8 years. She has a bachelor of arts degree in psychology and a master's degree in social work. She has worked as an early childhood special education teacher, a social worker in an early intervention program before the implementation of Part H, and as a training and technical assistance specialist with the Wisconsin Personnel Development Project. Ms. Irwin also participated in early intervention as a foster parent. She is especially interested in changing systems to be more responsive to families.

FOREWORD

◆ ◆ ◆

"Ok, ok, ok, I believe in these ideas, but what do I specifically do that is different?"

"Just because they passed a law with some letters and numbers, is that really going to make a big difference? You can't mandate sensitivity, and that is what is important."

The passage of early intervention legislation (i.e., Part H of PL 99-457, the Education of the Handicapped Act Amendments) in 1986 was revolutionary because of the law's emphasis on the importance of building collaborative relationships among families, professionals, disciplines, agencies, and institutions. The planning funds provided to states as a result of this legislation were sometimes described as "glue money," reflecting the intent that the funds be spent to develop strategies for integrating early intervention efforts across agencies, institutions, advocacy groups, disciplines, and constituents. The quotations above (one from a service provider and one from a parent) illustrate some of the frustrations and challenges that have accompanied the efforts of states, communities, and programs as they have moved from planning for family-centered, community-based approaches to early intervention to actual implementation of these plans. The challenges are twofold. The first challenge is how to translate the philosophical intent of Part H into actual practices. There are few professionals who would not espouse a family-centered approach; however, there are many different interpretations, some contradictory, about what such an approach means in terms of actual practices. The diversity in meanings and definitions, which, in part, legitimately reflect the diversity of early intervention programs and the families and communities served by those programs, leads to the second challenge: What are strategies for providing both experienced and entry-level professionals with information and skills related to building collaborative partnerships, and how can this information be used to help programs and the individuals associated with those programs (e.g., service providers, administrators, families) create their own unique collaborative relationships? No comprehensive text has addressed these challenges.

Partnerships in Family-Centered Care: A Guide to Collaborative Early Intervention meets the need for such a text with several unique features. Most available texts present information on family-centered, early intervention approaches by addressing the law, policies, and philosophy. This volume integrates and translates information about the law, policies, and philosophy into practical, day-to-day early intervention strategies related to building partnerships with families, teams, and agencies. This practical focus is reflected in the case studies, activities, and discussion questions that give the information real-world applications. This approach is particularly effective because it makes the information relevant to all disciplines and provides the trainer (or teacher) with material that generates in-depth discussion about early intervention practices with trainees of varied experience levels, disciplines, and settings. This volume is a particularly valuable training tool for interprofessional audiences; the discussions stimulated by the activities and case studies provide trainees, particularly preservice students, with opportunities to disagree with colleagues and to confront differences of opinion in the safety of the classroom. Experiences with such discussions are an important component of any training program.

A second unique feature of this text is the consistency of philosophy and integration of information across the chapters of the book. Strategies for collaboration with families, colleagues, and institutions share common features. The authors are able to build on information from previous chapters in a synthesizing fashion; at the same time, each chapter can stand alone, thoroughly addressing its particular content focus. This particular strength is undoubtedly a reflection of the fact that the authors themselves are an interprofessional team who have worked together for 5 years developing and implementing model demonstration and training programs in early intervention. As a team of individuals who represent allied health, early childhood special education, social work, and families, they have developed and articulated an integrated, consistent, and inclusive definition of family-centered, interdisciplinary practices. Together the authors are an effective model of what they espouse in their book, and this is evident in the integrated and consistent philosophy that permeates the volume.

This book represents a milestone for those teaching and practicing in early intervention. It takes a step in ensuring that partnerships among families, professionals, and agencies will develop and be nurtured by individuals who have a clear conception of what that means.

Pamela J. Winton, Ph.D.
Frank Porter Graham Child Development Center
University of North Carolina
Chapel Hill

PREFACE ◆◆◆

The passage of PL 99-457, the Education of the Handicapped Act Amendments, in 1986 and the changes made in 1991 when Part H of the law was reauthorized as PL 102-119, the Individuals with Disabilities Education Act (IDEA) Amendments, revolutionized the provision of services for infants and toddlers with special needs and their families. Those two important legislative mandates demanded changes in early intervention philosophy and practice.

IDEA (the name now used to refer comprehensively to legislation regarding the education of people with disabilities) now asks service providers to step outside of their traditional disciplinary roles as they provide family-centered services in a time when resources are scarce. Service providers are now charged with working closely with others in interdisciplinary, transdisciplinary, and interagency teams to coordinate services with families so that the outcomes of individualized family service plans (IFSPs) are met. Many service providers needed to learn new ways of working with families and with each other. This book's emphasis is on the knowledge and skills needed to serve as a foundation for service providers across all disciplines related to early intervention.

THE DEVELOPMENT OF THIS BOOK

This book originated from the Wisconsin Family-Centered Inservice Project (WFCIP). The 3-year (1990–1993) federally funded project (supported by the Office of Special Education and Rehabilitative Services) prepared personnel to meet the early intervention challenges resulting from IDEA's mandates. Specifically, the project addressed issues regarding the provision of *family-centered, interdisciplinary, coordinated services* to infants and toddlers with disabilities and their families.

The WFCIP in-service course and materials focused on cross-disciplinary information, issues, and strategies. General content areas featured were family-centered care, interdisciplinary and interagency teaming, and service coordination. The content and activities developed as part of WFCIP were field tested and refined through a series of for-credit university courses and various in-service formats. In addition, WFCIP benefited from the input of advisory committees composed of parents, service providers, agency personnel, and faculty. During the final 2 years of the project, the course content and activities were used to develop a volume entitled *Partnerships in Early Intervention: A Guide to Family-Centered Care, Team Building, and Service Coordination.* The guide was well received by in-service trainers and an interdisciplinary, early intervention faculty.

Based on the experiences of WFCIP, the content of the earlier volume, and the feedback from its audience, this book was written. It is intended for a wider audience than the earlier volume. This book is meant to be helpful to all service providers who work with infants and toddlers with special needs and their families. It is appropriate for use by professionals providing in-service training for health, education, and social services personnel. Such trainers may be associated with hospitals, clinics, agencies, direct services programs, or public schools. The book can also be used by faculty from a variety of departments on college and university campuses as the information and activities herein are appropriate for interdisciplinary or individual departmental courses.

THE CONTENT AND ORGANIZATION OF THIS BOOK

At the heart of this book are three interrelated themes: issues related to family-centered care, team building, and service coordination. Each chapter features a story, which is intended to facilitate independent and creative problem solving on issues raised throughout the chapter. The characters and situations presented in the stories serve as examples and illustrations to support the chapters' objectives.

This volume is divided into three sections. Section I, which includes Chapters 1–4, focuses on the philosophy and practices of family-centered care and various strategies for building partnerships between parents and service providers. Chapter 1 encourages readers to evaluate their own values as part of a process of working toward culturally sensitive and responsive services. Chapter 2 then provides up-to-date information about family systems—the broader context in which early intervention services are provided. In Chapter 3 the nature of the relationships developed in early intervention are explored. Reasons for partnership building are elucidated, and strategies for working toward partnerships are outlined. This section concludes with Chapter 4, which describes the IFSP process and stresses strategies for working in partnership.

The interdisciplinary and interagency teams of early intervention service provision are addressed in Section II. Chapter 5 discusses the types and purposes of teams and the roles that team members play. The underlying elements important to successful team functioning are the focus of Chapter 6, and Chapter 7 defines collaboration and discusses the benefits, challenges, and methods of working collaboratively.

The first three chapters in Section III emphasize service coordination. Chapter 8 describes current approaches to coordinating services, and Chapter 9 explores the functions and responsibilities one has as a service coordinator. Chapter 10 then identifies the elements of transition and provides strategies service coordinators and other early intervention personnel can use to support families during the transition process. Finally, Chapter 11 provides an overview of the historical development of the early intervention field. From this perspective, this chapter addresses the importance of parent–professional partnerships and interagency collaboration in shaping early intervention policy and practice. The chapter concludes by identifying a series of challenges facing the field of early intervention as it moves into the 21st century.

CONCLUSION

Successful family-centered early intervention has partnership as a foundation. Throughout the book, concepts, issues, and strategies are explored for working in partnership with others, including family members or other professionals. Being competent in early intervention means understanding and practicing many fundamental communication, decision-making, and conflict-managing skills. It involves listening, taking others' perspectives, and creating options and alternatives in arriving at solutions. Although this book highlights partnership as a central theme, it does not mean to downplay the importance of understanding new information about Part H regulations, the specifics of the IFSP and all its timelines, rights and procedural safeguards, and knowledge about the statewide and local service delivery systems. The goal of early intervention is to support families in a respectful way that is responsive to their needs for themselves and their children. If readers come closer to meeting this goal as a result of the ideas and activities presented and the discussions this text is intended to promote, we will have reached our aim in writing this book.

REFERENCES

Education of the Handicapped Act Amendments of 1986, PL 99-457. (October 8, 1986). Title 20, U.S.C. 1400 et seq: *U.S. Statutes at Large, 100,* 1145–1177.

Individuals with Disabilities Education Act Amendments of 1991, PL 102-119. (October 7, 1991). Title 20, U.S.C. 1400 et seq: *U.S. Statutes at Large, 105,* 587–608.

Rosin, P., Whitehead, A., Tuchman, L., Jesien, G., & Begun, A. (1993). *Partnerships in early intervention: A training guide on family-centered care, team building, and service coordination, Waisman Center, University of Wisconsin.* Madison: Wisconsin Family-Centered Inservice Project.

ACKNOWLEDGMENTS ◆ ◆ ◆

We wish to express our gratitude to all of the families who taught us what early intervention is and should be and who helped shape the vision underlying this book. We also thank the many reviewers and the advisory committee members whose input and feedback helped us to clarify this book's purpose and content; the faculty and students who participated in the Wisconsin Family-Centered Inservice Project; and Christopher Guadian, whose administrative assistance kept us organized. Finally and especially, we thank our own families, who patiently provided support and allowed us the time to put this book on paper.

PARTNERSHIPS IN FAMILY-CENTERED CARE

◆ ◆ ◆

I

FAMILY-CENTERED CARE
*Building Partnerships Between
Parents and Service Providers*

◆◆◆

1

THE DIVERSE AMERICAN FAMILY

Peggy Rosin

◆◆◆

OBJECTIVES

◆◆◆

By completing this chapter, the reader will

- Understand the concept of diversity and its importance in providing effective family-centered early intervention services
- Become aware of trends toward increasing cultural, structural, and socioeconomic diversity among families and the increasing number of parents with disabilities in the United States
- Recognize the barriers that may prevent some families from using early intervention services
- Understand the implications of family diversity for recommended practices in early intervention ◆

Throughout American history, the population of the United States has been among the most diverse in the world. The United States is a constantly changing mosaic of ethnic groups, religions, and socioeconomic classes. Diversity has challenged each generation of U.S. citizens to live up to national ideals of tolerance, fairness, and equal opportunity.

As the 21st century approaches, children and families in the United States are in transition. According to the National Commission on Children (1991), dramatic demographic, social, and economic changes have transformed the meaning of *family* in the United States. Four sources of diversity offer particular challenges in early intervention. First, growing numbers of families seeking early intervention services come from ethnic and cultural backgrounds that are different from those of many early intervention service providers. Second, structural changes in families mean that fewer children live in two-parent families with mothers who are full-time homemakers. Third, the number of infants and toddlers living in poverty is increasing. And fourth, the number of families with parents with disabilities is growing.

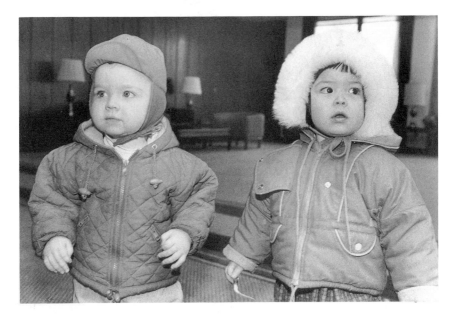

Policies and programs designed to meet the mandates of Part H of the Individuals with Disabilities Education Act (IDEA) of 1990, PL 101-476, are being developed in the midst of these changes. The intent of Part H is to develop a service delivery system with families as the focal point, serving as partners and decision makers in the early intervention process. Family-centered services are based on principles that stress respect for family diversity. Several principles suggested by McGonigel, Johnson, and Kaufmann (1991) are related to family diversity.

- States and programs should define *family* in a way that reflects the diversity of family patterns and structures.
- Each family has its own structure, roles, values, beliefs, and coping styles. Respect for and acceptance of family diversity is a cornerstone of family-centered early intervention.
- Early intervention systems and strategies must honor the racial, ethnic, cultural, and socioeconomic diversity of families.

When the U.S. Congress passed the Individuals with Disabilities Education Act Amendments of 1991, PL 102-119, it amended the law to clearly define states' obligations to low-income and minority families. Beginning in 1992, states must

> provide satisfactory assurance that policies and practices have been adopted to ensure meaningful involvement of traditionally underserved groups, including minority, low-income, and rural families, in the planning and implementation of all the requirements of this part and to ensure that such families have access to culturally competent services within their local areas. (Senate Bill 1106, Section 678b)

Cultural competence refers to attitudes, actions, and policies of individuals, agencies, and systems. Cultural competence is "a program's ability to honor and respect those beliefs, interpersonal styles, attitudes, and behaviors both of families who are clients and the multicultural staff who are providing services" (Roberts, 1990, p. 1). This chapter provides introductory information regarding diversity, as well as a framework and suggestions for service providers and early intervention programs in working toward cultural competence. The chapter stresses that the attitudes and processes that help one move toward cultural competence are similar to those needed by service providers in working with families who may differ from practitioners in a number of respects (e.g., socioeconomic status, family structure, parents who have disabilities).

SHEILA SHANAHAN'S STORY

Sheila Shanahan has been a speech-language pathologist for 5 years. She thinks of herself as a knowledgeable and caring professional who tries to do her best. She has just accepted a position at a large, urban early intervention program.

Sheila believes that she is well informed about the typical and atypical development of communication skills in infants and toddlers. But she knows her experience in working with families is limited. She has provided information to parents regarding testing of their children that she has completed, and she has suggested ways for parents to facilitate their children's communication. Her training, however, has not addressed working with families.

Sheila grew up in a large, Anglo-European, middle-class, two-parent family in northern Wisconsin. She attended parochial schools through college and went to graduate school in Wisconsin. She realizes that she has spent most of her life surrounded by people with backgrounds similar to her own, but she does not yet fully appreciate the challenges of her new position.

By the end of her first month on the job, Sheila knew that she had much to learn about other people, their values, and their lifestyles. She wants to become more knowledgeable about the diverse families with whom she is working in the individualized family service plan (IFSP) process. She has attended some workshops about the state's birth-to-3 initiative, but these have focused on the general principles of family-centered services. Sheila wants to develop new skills that will help her build partnerships with families, especially those whose values and experiences differ from her own.

Today is a fairly typical day for Sheila. She is part of the evaluation team that determines infants' and toddlers' eligibility for early intervention services. The team is meeting with a Hmong family and their twins,

Bao and Dao. The twins were born in the United States; however, their parents, Mr. and Mrs. Xiang, refugees from northern Laos, have been in the United States for only 3 years. Their knowledge of English is quite limited. Sheila has thoroughly read the available medical and diagnostic records on the children, who are now 2 years old. These records give a clear picture of the children's development.

What the records do not reveal are the questions and concerns Mr. and Mrs. Xiang may have about their children. Sheila and the other team members hope that the family will feel comfortable enough at today's meeting to share some of those questions and concerns. Sheila understands that an interpreter from the Hmong community will accompany the Xiang family today. She knows that she needs to organize her conversation with the Xiangs so that she can help them to talk about their hopes and dreams for their children, their immediate and long-term priorities and concerns, and the resources available to them. Sheila also wants to find out how the Xiangs would like to be involved in their children's evaluation and in possible subsequent IFSP meetings.

WORKING TOWARD CULTURAL COMPETENCE

Sheila's story is not uncommon among service providers in early intervention. Across many health, educational, and social services disciplines working with infants and toddlers with disabilities and their families, there has been a paucity of training related to families, especially families who differ from the "mainsteam" American family (Christensen, 1992; Vergara, 1992). There is no doubt that the notion of mainstream America is changing and needs to be changed in light of the diverse families who comprise American society. In Sheila's story we find a service provider struggling to secure skills essential for working with families in a culturally competent manner.

How can Sheila gain the competence she needs in interacting with families with backgrounds different from her own? In a conceptual model formulated by Christensen (1989), cross-cultural awareness is viewed as a developmental task for all people that involves the discovery and integration "of the personal and sociopolitical meaning of one's ethnicity, culture, and race as these affect oneself and others" (p. 274). Therefore, one can think of Sheila's movement toward cultural competence as a process, not a trait. Movement toward cultural competence is incremental, with each stage distinguished from the others by the person's level of awareness about other cultures. Sheila can assess her own developmental stage of cross-cultural awareness and can in turn apply strategies to promote her transition to the next stage of cross-cultural awareness. In moving toward cultural competence, stages may need to be revisited as service providers confront new cultural groups or values and lifestyles with which they are not familiar.

A variety of approaches for achieving cultural competence have been suggested (Chan, 1990; Christensen, 1989; Lynch & Hanson, 1992, 1993; Yacobacci-Tam, 1987). When similar elements from a number of approaches are integrated, a process emerges that allows Sheila and other service providers a means of acquiring knowledge and skills to work with diverse families.

The process of working toward cultural competence begins with exploring one's own culture and understanding how one's background is the foundation upon which relationships with families are formed. The next step in the process is gaining information about sources of diversity. The third step is examining possible barriers faced by families when obtaining early intervention services. The fourth step is developing strategies to help service providers and programs build partnerships with a wide variety of families.

Step #1: Exploring One's Own Culture

Culture shapes every person's life. Cunningham, Cunningham, and O'Connell (1986) have stated

> Culture is now known to be a people's traditional values, beliefs, and behaviors. Values are defined as that which is held to be important. Beliefs are that which are held to be true. Behaviors are patterns of daily activities. An understanding of culture includes how values and beliefs are given form in people's lives. (p. 3)

It is essential for service providers to understand how their own values, beliefs, and behaviors influence their interactions with and responses to families.

This form of cultural self-analysis is integral to numerous guidelines suggested for service providers working to gain cross-cultural competence (Chan, 1990; Lynch & Hanson, 1993; Harry, 1992; Lynch, 1992; Patterson & Blum, 1993; Ramer, 1992; Yacobacci-Tam, 1987). The following self-assessment strategies are offered to assist service providers like Sheila in thinking about their own cultural values.

Strategy: Comparing Your Values to American and Western Values

Yacobacci-Tam (1987) has proposed a process to develop cross-cultural understanding. One stage of her process entails analyzing one's own personal beliefs and values in relation to the American and Western culture that pervades the service delivery system. Table 1.1 outlines several contrasting cultural values.

Cultural traditions affect how people act and interact in response to life experiences. This includes how service providers in early intervention conduct their practices. For example, some people raised in the American and Western culture may value a spirit of competition. Their early experiences may have stressed achievement through competition in sports and education. This in turn may influence how such service

Table 1.1. Contrasting cultural values

Eastern culture	American and Western culture
Being	Doing
Family/group/community emphasis	Individual emphasis, privacy
Interdependence	Independence
Cooperation	Competition
Person-to-person orientation	Person-to-object orientation
Authoritarian orientation	Democratic orientation
Hierarchy, rank, status	Egalitarianism
Extended family	Nuclear family, blended family
Rigid family member roles	Flexible family member roles
Favoritism toward males	Increasing female role
Formality	Informality
Indirectness, ritual, face	Directness, openness, honesty
Suppression of emotions	Expression of emotions
Fate	Mastery of one's own future
Balance and harmony, tradition	Change
Patience, modesty	Assertiveness
Personal interaction dominant	Time dominant
Spiritualism, detachment	Materialism
Birthright and inheritance	Self-help
Past orientation	Future orientation
"Being" orientation	Action, goal, work orientation
Idealism and theory	Practicality and efficiency

Adapted by permission from Kohls, L.R. (1984). *The values Americans live by.* Washington, DC: Meridian International Center (1630 Crescent Place, N.W., Washington, DC 20009; [202] 667-6800).

providers participate on various transdisciplinary or interagency teams. Working collaboratively on early intervention teams (i.e., holding common goals, sharing resources, ensuring equal participation) may be contrary to the service providers' experience of team competition. In this example, it is essential to examine how a sense of competitiveness could interfere with a team's tasks and to determine whether behaviors need to be modified for more effective team membership.

The importance one places on time, promptness, and adherence to schedules is another example of a value that influences interactions in early intervention settings. If a family's or caregiver's values are consistent with those associated with the American and Western culture (i.e., that time dominates), but the service provider values personal interaction over being on time for a scheduled appointment, the possibility for conflict arises. The service provider may run overtime in an earlier appointment and arrive late to meet the family who values promptness. If tardiness on the part of the service provider is habitual, it can be a source of conflict between the family and that provider.

Strategy: Storytelling to Reflect on Personal Values

Telling stories about one's personal experiences and listening to the stories of others (e.g., families, co-workers, service providers from various agencies) can be a powerful way to reflect upon how culture permeates everyone's actions and beliefs.

> In universities people know through studies. In business and bureaucracies, people know by reports. In communities, people know by stories. These community stories allow people to reach back into their individual experience for knowledge about truth and direction for the future. (McKnight, 1995, p. 9)

Remember that working toward being culturally competent service providers entails continual self-assessment of cultural values. The following activity provides an opportunity for self-reflection through storytelling and addressing the questions related to storytelling.

ACTIVITY:

◆ ◆ ◆

Exploring Values Through Storytelling

Explore your own values by choosing one value listed on Table 1.1 and telling a story to a colleague or friend that illustrates the value's influence on your life.

How does it feel to share your values through a story?
Do you think it useful in exploring your own cultural values?
How might stories be used in working with families in early intervention? ◆

Strategy: Exploring Stereotypes

Campt (1992) and McCormack (1987) have advised service providers to examine their attitudes regarding stereotypic views (i.e., beliefs about groups of individuals) and ethnocentrism (i.e., belief in the superiority of one's own culture). Pinderhughes (1988) reported that there may be active, yet repressed, feelings that interfere with successful cross-cultural counseling. Among Anglo-European counselors, these feelings could include guilt, anxiety, fear, self-doubt, and a desire to protect ethnic groups. Determining whether one holds stereotypic views about particular groups and exploring the basis for these stereotypic views may be important before working with representatives of these groups. A potentially safe way to gain knowledge and ask questions about cultural groups and issues is to attend classes, workshops, and discussions about cultural diversity.

Strategy: Taking a Cultural Journey

Lynch (1992) suggests that service providers embark on a "cultural journey" to explore and discuss their origins, beliefs, biases, and behaviors.

On the journey the service provider imagines life from the perspectives of people from different ethnic backgrounds.

Step #2: Understanding Sources of Family Diversity

In Step #2, the service provider seeks information about the diverse families with whom he or she works, compares the findings to his or her own cultural self-analysis, and attempts to reconcile differences. This increased sensitivity to families with a variety of backgrounds is the basis for developing skills and modifying practices that respect diverse families.

Of course, each family is unique and must be approached individually. A family may belong to a particular socioeconomic or cultural group or have a certain lifestyle, but these facts should not become the basis for stereotypical assumptions.

> We recognize the danger of generalizing. We know that there is great diversity within any group. General statements about a group have the potential to reinforce harmful stereotypes. But general awareness also has the power to build respect for cultures rooted in representations of reality that unfold from conditions different from our own. (Edmunds, Martinson, & Goldberg, 1990, p. 1)

With these cautions in mind, the following section briefly discusses sources of diversity within the American family.

Cultural Diversity

A culturally distinct population may be defined as a group of people with a shared identity determined by common racial or ethnic origins, languages, customs, and religions. Such people share complex patterns of behavior derived from common knowledge, beliefs, goals, perceptions, customs, and values. Culture has a dramatic influence on a family by shaping its values, structure, functions, development, and adaptation. Culture affects interaction among family members and between the family and the larger community.

Understanding one's own cultural values is stressed in the first step of moving toward cultural competence. Equally important is understanding how each family defines itself or identifies with its culture. Culture is mediated by differing degrees of acculturation, socioeconomic and educational status, occupation, and geographic factors. It is crucial that the early intervention system avoid defining families according to cultural, ethnic, gender, or socioeconomic generalizations or stereotypes. At the same time, information about a family's culture can help the practitioner explore with family members their values and preferences regarding use of early intervention services. Such information can help the service provider to acknowledge and respect cultural differences and to serve the family more effectively.

Demographers predict that a century from now the racial makeup of the U.S. population will more closely resemble that of the entire world, in which 57% of people are Asian, 26% are Anglo-European, and 7% are African (National Commission on Children, 1991). People of Hispanic origin—11% of the U.S. population in 1989—can be of any race. By the year 2010, nearly 25% of all children in the United States will be children of color. The Hispanic and Asian populations have grown especially rapidly since the mid-1980s. This makes it essential that early intervention service providers and programs become increasingly culturally competent by gaining information about families with cultures different from their own.

Strategy: Reviewing Written Information

The literature is replete with summaries of commonalities found among cultural and ethnic groups, including African Americans, Native Americans, Anglo-Europeans, Asian Americans, and Hispanics (Hanline & Daley, 1992; Kanemoto, 1987; Krajewski-Jaime, 1991; Leung, 1988; Locust, 1985; Lynch & Hanson, 1992; McCubbin, Thompson, Thompson, McCubbin, & Kaston, 1993; Morrow, 1987). As a prelude to their discussion of the acceptance of disability in the Mexican American culture, Smart and Smart (1991) caution readers that conclusions drawn from the literature may 1) unduly focus on a subgroup of the cultural and/or ethnic group, 2) fail to separate the effects of culture from the effects of socioeconomic factors, 3) fail to keep abreast of rapid demographic changes, and 4) rely too heavily on survey methods of research. These cautions may apply in reviewing the literature about all groups.

Lynch and Hanson (1992) have provided an extensive synthesis of cultural perspectives related to geographic, religious, and linguistic origins, as well as to contemporary lifestyles, values, and beliefs. This synthesis is intended expressly for the early interventionist to gain basic information regarding major cultural groups. Understanding others' cultural perspectives can have a tremendous impact on practices in early intervention. For example, Krajewski-Jaime (1991) discusses the importance of understanding the validity and integrity of folk-healing interventions for some Mexican Americans. Without considering the cultural contexts of some folk-healing practices, some service providers may interpret decisions not to follow recommended treatments as ignorance, superstition, neglect, or abuse.

ACTIVITY: *Getting Culturally Specific Information*

◆ ◆ ◆

Reflect on Sheila's situation: What information might Sheila want to know about the Hmong people before meeting with Mr. and Mrs. Xiang that would be useful to her in communicating with them about their children and the IFSP process?   ◆

Strategy: Become Familiar with the Community's Formal and Informal Supports

One way to extend one's knowledge about a particular community is to become familiar with those whom the community looks to for information and support. Ask questions about whether there are community leaders and social, religious, and/or political groups from which the community receives support. Informal discussions with community leaders and others in the community can help to increase general knowledge about the needs and networks of the people receiving services in the community. Publications such as newspapers, newsletters, or magazines that are read frequently by community members may be sources of information. If appropriate, attend holiday celebrations, special events, or community meetings.

In establishing relationships with families of different cultures, ethnographic information may be useful. It may be most appropriate to request such information from a community spokesperson or an agency familiar with the culture. The kinds of information that may be helpful include the following:

- *Group description*—country of origin, language, dialect, and number of people of that ethnic group in the local area
- *Social organization in the community*—informal and formal supports used by community members in the local area and the roles of community leaders

It will also be important to know the level of acculturation of the family into the majority culture. Some families, known as *mainstreamers*, prefer to identify themselves as Americans and become part of the majority culture as much as possible. *Culturally contained* families take pride in their cultural traditions and associate primarily with others of similar backgrounds. Still others are bicultural, associating with members of the majority culture as well as with their own ethnic group. Knowing where the family is on the cultural continuum assists in determining how and where services might best be provided. For example, the service provider might thus be prompted to ask the family whether an interpreter, advocate, community leader, or anyone else should be included in meetings and decision making.

Structural Diversity

Many Americans perceive of the traditional family as comprising an employed father, a homemaker mother, and children, all of whom live under one roof. In fact, that profile describes only 7% of families in the United States. In 1989, 25% of all American children were living with only one of their parents, most often the mother (National Commission on Children, 1991). An expanding rate of divorce and increasing births to unmarried women account for the rising number of single-parent families. Blended families or stepfamilies, including children from prior relationships of one or both parents, are also becoming more common. Moreover, mothers, whether married or single, are far more likely to be employed outside the home than they were a generation ago. Between 1970 and 1990, the proportion of mothers with children under 6 years old in the paid work force increased from 32% to 58%.

Other changes in family structure cited by Hanson and Lynch (1992) include increased numbers of adoptive and foster families, parenting by grandparents or other extended family members, and same-sex parents. The Children's Defense Fund (1993) reported that an estimated 1.3 million children in the United States are cared for by grandparents or other relatives because the parents are not in the home. Often relatives are full-time caregivers for the children but do not have legal custody or guardianship. This becomes a complex issue when attempting to provide early intervention to families. These sources of structural diversity are widely debated with regard to their impact on children.

Living in Poverty

One in four children under the age of 3 years lives in poverty. Statistics reported by the National Center for Children in Poverty (1995) revealed that this disturbing trend is on the rise, and the number of poor children under the age of 6 years increased significantly. The association between low income and various negative outcomes for children is well documented (Brookins, 1993; Hanson & Lynch, 1992). Many children living in poverty are undernourished, live in substandard housing, experience health problems, and do not have access to adequate health care. Studies (e.g., Carnegie Corporation Task Force on Meeting the Needs of Young Children, 1994) estimate that of the approximately 100,000 American children who are homeless, about one half are under 6 years of age. Poverty can place children at risk for developmental problems. Resilience in the face of economic and social hardship is well documented but not well understood. Many families and children confronted with such challenges still are able to do well.

A disproportionate number of people of color in the United States live in poverty (National Commission on Children, 1991). Figure 1.1 shows that poverty rates are significantly greater for African American and Hispanic families, and that the trend is greatly exacerbated for young children living in single-parent families.

Parents with Disabilities

Families headed by parents with disabilities, whether physical, emotional, cognitive, or sensory, are becoming more common. Society, however, offers little emotional or financial support for the endeavor. "There is a need for studies that explore the strengths and weaknesses of parent-

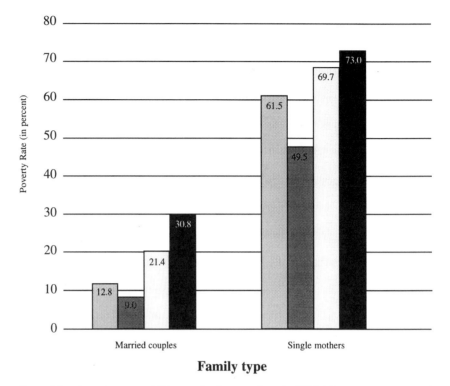

Figure 1.1.   Poverty among children under 3 years of age in 1990. Ninety-seven percent of all children under 3 years of age who live with single parents live with their mothers, and 3% live with their fathers. (From Einbinder, S.D. [1992]. *A statistical profile of children living in poverty: Children under three and children under six, 1990.* Unpublished manuscript, Columbia University School of Public Health, National Center for Children in Poverty, New York; reprinted by permission.)

ing by people with disabilities and research on when, where, and how much, if any, social support is needed" (Gray & Schimmel, 1993, p. 350).

There seems to be a consensus that parents with mental retardation are at risk for parenting practices that lead to referral to child protective services (Lynch & Bakley, 1989). Their parenting styles are often affected not only by their mental retardation but also by many associated factors (e.g., low income, poor housing, lack of transportation, isolation). Espe-Sherwindt and Crable (1993) encourage service providers to set aside myths about parents with mental retardation. They argue that providing support to parents with mental retardation can build competence and make a critical difference in their parenting.

Parents with physical disabilities—whether the disabilities are life-long, the result of accidents causing acquired brain injury, or due to disorders such as muscular dystrophy—may face obstacles to participation. Accessibility can be a major issue because of architectural hindrances, lack of transportation, communication problems, and lack of flexibility resulting from reliance on attendant care. For example, architectural barriers can prevent parents from participating in events planned for their child. One parent related that she was unable to attend a preschool screening with her child because it was held in a church basement. The idea was to save the district money on the screening location, but no one considered whether the location was accessible. Lack of transportation or dependence on specialized public or private transportation can cause scheduling and attendance difficulties. Also, for some parents with physical disabilities, speech can be affected by a motor disorder. This can result in difficulty communicating in person and, especially, by telephone. If the parent is reliant on assistive technology, it may not always be available, and if it is available it can be cumbersome and slow the interaction. Some parents with physical disabilities need to schedule their participation in conjunction with their attendant. This adds another level of complexity in scheduling and participation.

Limited research available on the subject suggests that, in general, parents with disabilities are as effective as parents without disabilities in their parenting roles. The numerous environmental and attitudinal barriers faced by people with disabilities, however, can have negative effects on their families, including their children.

Families with Multiple Challenges

It is important to remember that a family may be affected by more than one of the factors mentioned here and may face additional challenges as well. A family may be new to the United States, speak little or no English, live in poverty, and have little informal support. Another family may have a low income and be headed by a single parent with health problems such as drug and alcohol addiction. Benn (1993) cautions that although it is difficult to determine the effects of individual risk factors (e.g., parents' mental illness, homelessness, substance abuse) on a child's outcome, as risk factors multiply, the likelihood of these factors having an adverse effect on the child is increased.

The combination of challenges facing a family can be overwhelming. Therefore, it is imperative that the system function in a supportive and collaborative manner across agencies. For many families with multiple stresses, there are often multiple agencies (e.g., medical, social, legal) with which they may need to interact to meet their needs. Sometimes for families in stress, having to negotiate multiple agencies can add to, rather than alleviate, stress. A system that is flexible and adaptable can be more responsive to families. It is critical for the early intervention service coordinator to consider an entire family's needs and to work in concert with other agency personnel to ensure that the family is receiving appropriate services and support.

Step #3: Understanding the Barriers to Using Early Intervention Services

Anderson and Schrag Fenichel (1989) state that "the effectiveness of programs to provide services for multicultural populations of infants and toddlers with disabilities and their families rests heavily upon the sensitivity, understanding, and respect paid to specific cultural, familial, and individual diversity involved" (p. 18). But others have argued that acknowledgment, awareness, and good intentions are not sufficient to produce culturally and linguistically appropriate services. Strategies must be developed to remove the barriers that many families encounter in trying to use health, educational, and social services.

Medical, educational, and social services systems tend to develop policies and procedures that meet the needs of organizations rather than the needs of the people they serve. Even conscious efforts by such organizations to meet people's needs are often limited by the assumption that consumers have the same preferences, needs, resources, and values as the people working for the organization. Such assumptions create barriers to other people's use of the services (Condeluci, 1991).

Careful study and application of a family-centered paradigm can help early intervention programs be truly responsive to the needs of families. Each family's needs are unique and must receive individual consideration. Awareness of the kinds of barriers encountered frequently by families, especially those who differ in some way from the typical two-parent, Anglo-European, middle-class family for whom most programs are designed, can help professionals to examine their own attitudes and behaviors and their organizations' policies and procedures.

Lack of Understanding of Differences in Values and Customs

Values differ from one culture to the next. When cultural values are not understood and respected, misunderstandings occur (Campt, 1992; Leung, 1988; Morrow, 1987; Turner, 1987). Both parties may feel uncomfortable. A family whose values are not understood by a service provider may decide not to continue the relationship. Table 1.1 lists contrasting values that can lead to misunderstandings and conflicts among individuals, families, and cultures.

These differences have implications for all cross-cultural relationships. Their impact will reverberate throughout the IFSP process as a family interacts with service providers. For example, people of some cultures often socialize children to live in the present, placing a higher value on completing social interactions than on adhering to a schedule. This can affect the way in which these individuals are viewed by people of other cultures who value punctuality and adherence to a schedule. Conflict may result, especially if one party is frequently late for appointments and the other is usually 5 minutes early.

Different cultures have different values and customs regarding issues directly related to early intervention, including children, childbearing and child rearing, family roles, disabilities, medicine and healing, language and communication, diet and nutrition, seeking help outside the family, and gender roles, among others. It is clear that values and customs regarding these issues will have an impact on relationships between families and early intervention service providers. For example, Hanson, Lynch, and Wayman (1990) reported that in some Asian cultures, physical closeness is more highly valued than vocal and verbal stimulation during the early years of life. Touch is the primary means of communication with the child. A speech-language pathologist, as in Sheila's story, might easily misinterpret the lack of parent–child verbal interaction, seeing it as requiring remediation when, in fact, it is a cultural characteristic. The service provider's misunderstanding of the family's culture thus would present a barrier to an effective relationship.

Family roles, including who is viewed as the head of the household, how decisions are made within the family, who is seen as the primary caregiver, and the importance of the extended family in decision making, vary from culture to culture. The early intervention service provider must understand the roles and structure of each family, especially regarding decision making. The family members with key decision-making roles must be included in each meeting at which decisions are to be made.

Communication Barriers

Communication is the means by which values and beliefs are expressed. How service providers talk with families is the basis upon which partnerships are built or denied. All communication involves a delicate balance of reading and interpreting the verbal and nonverbal messages of the communicators. When communicating cross-culturally, the "dynamic of difference" may be most easily felt. Service providers in a multicultural society need to understand and be responsive to cultural differences while also not assuming that information about a culture applies to a specific family.

Several authors provide guidelines for service providers when communicating cross-culturally with different ethnic groups (Chan, Lam, Wong, Leung, & Fang, 1988; Marshall, Martin, Thomason, & Johnson, 1991; Matsuda, 1989; McCormack, 1987). For example, Matsuda (1989) offered the following eight guidelines for communicating effectively with Asian families: 1) be status conscious, 2) try to reach consensus on recommendations, 3) be pragmatic, 4) respect cultural beliefs and incorporate them into intervention, 5) use indirect approaches, 6) be patient and quiet, 7) be informative, and 8) pay attention to nonverbal cues. Orlansky and Trapp (1987) suggested guidelines for communicating with Native Americans, including the following: 1) do not expect direct eye contact, 2) do not probe deeply, 3) develop a tolerance for silence, 4) do not reprimand or praise a Native American person in front of others, 5) shake hands gently, 6) use demonstrations of actual skills or technqiues, 7) be sensitive to the person's perception of time and scheduling, 8) respect the importance of the extended family, and 9) avoid stereotypes and generalizations. It must be stated emphatically, however, that these are general guidelines and should not be applied across the board in all circumstances. Thomason (1991) stated that some Native Americans are offended by the idea that the suggestions of Orlansky and Trapp (1987) apply to them, and suggested that individual behaviors, such as tone of voice, pace of speech, and eye contact, be noted and subtly matched.

Some barriers to communication are far less subtle than those caused by different values and customs. Some families do not speak English. Some do not read, at least not well enough to understand forms and notices they receive in the mail. Parents who are deaf may need an interpreter if the people with whom they interact do not know sign language. Parents with visual impairments may need materials in a large-print format or on cassette.

It often takes longer for families with special communication needs to learn that early intervention programs exist, because the usual ways of publicizing such programs are not understandable to them. Developing relationships with key people in the cultural groups of the local area can help to create an awareness of early intervention services in the community.

Financial Barriers

Even when there is no charge for early intervention services, there may be *associated costs* that present barriers to participation for families, especially those with limited informal or financial supports. Transportation to an early intervention program, child care for other offspring, and unpaid time off from work to attend meetings are examples of associated costs. Early intervention programs can make it easier for parents to participate by helping with these costs. (e.g., paying for transportation to early intervention services, including siblings in the intervention when appropriate, arranging meeting times that will accomodate the parents' work schedules).

Effects of Past Experience

Some families have had bad prior experiences with health care, educational, or human services systems. Such experiences may lead families to expect the worst from early intervention. Red tape, bureaucratic delays and insensitivity, and a tendency to blame service recipients are, unfortunately, not uncommon.

Each ethnic group has a history from which its cultural traditions develop. Current relations between ethnic groups should be viewed in light of their historical contexts. For example, the historical treatment of

Native Americans (Toubbeh, 1985) and African Americans in the United States affects these groups' level of trust in today's society and in its institutions. Racism and discrimination are not just old memories. A family member confronted with discrimination shares these experiences with the rest of his or her family. These experiences are recounted among family members and passed on from generation to generation. Building trust in the system and in its representatives is predicated upon replacing old, negative stories with new, positive ones.

Scheduling Barriers

Almost all families with infants and toddlers are busy families. For single-parent families and families in which both parents work, demands on time are particularly great. Responding to individual families' scheduling needs will make it easier for them to participate.

Step #4: Developing Culturally Competent Early Intervention Services

Cultural competence extends beyond individual service providers to the early intervention programs and the multiple health, educational, and social services systems in which families are involved. A program or system moves toward cultural competence by entering a process similar to the one described for service providers. In Step #4, the service provider is encouraged to look at the early intervention programs and systems in which he or she works and evaluate and promote cultural competence in all policies and procedures. Five essential elements should be reflected in a culturally competent program. These elements include 1) valuing diversity, 2) promoting cultural self-assessment, 3) acknowledging the dynamics inherent in cultural interactions, 4) institutionalizing cultural knowledge, and 5) adapting to diversity (Cross, Bazron, Dennis, & Isaacs, 1989).

Many programs may need to modify existing policies and procedures to reflect cultural sensitivity. Roberts (1990), in association with colleagues, developed the *Workbook for Developing Culturally Competent Programs*, which provides programs with a series of self-study questions. These questions assist programs to examine policies and practices for providing culturally competent services.

Rogler, Malgady, Costantino, and Blumenthal (1987) discussed three broad approaches for increasing cultural sensitivity in mental health services. The three approaches can be viewed as a pyramid. At the base are programs that attempt to increase the accessibility of services to certain populations. In the middle are programs that choose treatments according to the cultural characteristics of a certain group. At the top are programs that are modified according to an understanding and evaluation of ethnic characteristics. Service providers are encouraged to adapt their services for culturally distinct populations into this pyramidal structure and to conduct research that evaluates the efficacy of these approaches.

One example of an early intervention program designed to provide culturally sensitive early intervention services to families of Puerto Rican heritage was described by Bruder, Anderson, Schutz, and Caldera (1991). To meet this goal, program components of the 3-year model demonstration project, *Niños Especiales*, were tailored to promote culturally competent services consistent with the characteristics of the top level of services described by Rogler et al. (1987). Based on their project evaluation, Bruder and colleagues suggested that several general modifications be made in program services provided for Puerto Rican families. These modifications include 1) providing adequate bilingual services for the family; 2) promoting awareness of the Puerto Rican culture and how it may differ from the U.S. culture in terms of family relationships, child-rearing practices, support networks, societal responsibilities, social etiquette, and belief in fate; and 3) preparing and training staff to be responsive to family-identified needs.

Zuniga (1992) provides excellent resource suggestions for working with Latino families. She emphasizes that each Latino family should be viewed individually, but she also identifies cultural themes relevant to how programs for the Latino population might be modified. For example, courtesies for the service provider to consider during interactions with Latino families include 1) accepting food or beverage if they are offered; 2) beginning with a relaxed, informal tone before getting down to the task at hand; and 3) using an unhurried manner.

WORKING WITH DIVERSE FAMILIES IN THE IFSP PROCESS

To a certain extent, early intervention programs can reduce barriers to diverse families' participation in the IFSP process through changes in policies and procedures. But for each family, the combination of barriers and incentives will be unique. In getting to know a family, a service provider must be aware of differences in cultural values and individual resources, as well as of other barriers discussed previously, so that these can be addressed. Knowing a family's cultural background, structure, or economic level can help service providers to shape appropriate services for that family. It must be stressed, however, that individual families have their own characteristics that may or may not reflect what is considered typical for a particular ethnic group, family structure, or socioeconomic class.

Building a Relationship

Being Culturally Sensitive

There are special considerations when building a cross-cultural relationship. The service provider must know him- or herself (i.e., be aware of his or her attitudes, values, and priorities), must know about the general characteristics of the culture of the family with whom he or she is working (e.g., history, geography, language, religion, views about child-rearing roles), must understand possible barriers for the family when gaining access to services, and must modify existing program policies and procedures to be relevant and accessible to the family.

Communication Considerations

The IFSP process begins with initial contact with the family. Therefore, the service provider must be sensitive to possible differences in communication styles from the first conversation with the family. Communication differences may be apparent in both verbal and nonverbal interactions. Different ethnic groups interpret nonverbal cues, such as body language, silence, pauses, proximity between speakers, eye contact, and emotional or facial expressions, in different ways. For example, many Anglo-Europeans feel uncomfortable after a pause of several seconds during a conversation and will end the pause. For some Native Americans, however, a minute may be a typical amount of time to take in responding.

Verbal communication styles also differ across cultures. Service providers should become aware of how they use their voices (i.e., rate, volume, inflection) to impart respect and assist listeners in understanding. Formality should be monitored. One family may appreciate an informal tone, and this style may enhance rapport with them. Another family may find formality to be offensive. For example, some African Americans prefer to be addressed as Mr. or Ms. Use of their first names by people who do not know them well is viewed as disrespectful.

Similarly, families may think of certain topics as private. Their values should be respected. They should be assured that they do not need to address any topic or answer any question that makes them uncomfortable.

For some families, English is a second language. Therefore, it is important to avoid slang, technical jargon, and complex sentences, especially if an interpreter is not present. Service providers should try to remember their experiences with a foreign language. If an interpreter is needed, he or she should be sure to address the family, not the interpreter. Open-ended questions may assist in gaining information. Lynch (1992) provides excellent suggestions and guidelines for working with interpreters.

First Contacts with Families: Interviewing and Asking Questions

An interview might be the service provider's first contact with a family and may be the first opportunity to share information and begin the process of building a partnership. The service provider acknowledges the family's resources and builds on the family's competence. Westby (1990) provides a model for interviewing that incorporates the effects of culture on participants and suggests specific methods for 1) building rapport, 2) using descriptive questions, and 3) wording questions carefully. Kalyanpur and Rao (1991) have found that being conversational; interpreting, sharing and offering strategies by telling stories from past experience; and accepting and supporting mothers' confidence about their skills as parents are ways to establish rapport when working with some African American families with low incomes.

Wayman, Lynch, and Hanson (1990) have provided guidelines for service providers as they begin working with the family, the most intimate of systems. They offer a series of questions as a tool for gathering information through conversations with the family. Each family's interests should guide the service provider in deciding which questions to ask. Of course, all the questions need not be asked or answered in the initial meeting. Information will be shared over time as a relationship develops between the family and the service provider. The information gained can be used in planning and providing services to the family. The questions are organized in the following three parts:

Family Structure and Child-Rearing Practices includes questions about family composition and primary caregiving for the child. The service provider might ask, "Who are important people in your child's life?" and "With whom does your child spend the day?" A "family portrait" could be drawn by asking who would be included in the picture. Additional questions ask about the family's child-rearing practices concerning feeding and mealtimes, sleeping patterns, and responding to the child's behavior. The service provider can use open-ended questions such as "Tell me" about how your baby eats, sleeps, or plays. If from the referral information or collateral data the service provider knows that there are parental concerns, he or she can ask the parent to "Tell me about your concerns" in a specific developmental area. If the parent acknowledges an area of concern in describing the child's behavior, it may be appropriate to probe further by asking more specific questions such as, "Where does the child eat?", "When does the child eat?", or "What are the child's favorite foods?"

Family Perceptions and Attitudes includes questions about the family's perception of their child's disability, their beliefs about health and healing, and how they feel about seeking help for themselves and their child. Here the service provider may ask parents to describe how they view their child's health and development. Questions may be asked about previous contacts (assessments, diagnoses) with other health, social services, or education agencies. The parents may describe their understanding of what others have said about their child's development and whether they are in agreement with these assessments.

Family Language and Interaction Style includes questions about the family's first language, English proficiency, and need for an interpreter. If the family does not use English as a primary language and the service provider does not speak the family's first language, the family should be asked if they want an interpreter made available to them or if they would like to invite someone they trust to interpret. Additional questions ask about their preference for receiving information (in writing, over the phone, in person) and their preference for how the service provider interacts with them during visits. For all families, a menu of options for receiving information should be offered.

When parents have disabilities, service providers need to ask about their preferences and needs. A parent who is blind may need to receive written information and have it read to her prior to a meeting. A parent who is deaf may need an interpreter. A parent with developmental disabilities or mental illness may want to bring a support person to meetings.

Low-income and ethnic families may be very alert to nonverbal communication. When visiting a family in their home, the service provider is a guest. A polite guest does not clutch her purse tightly throughout a visit or brush off a chair before sitting on it. Appropriate clothing is clean and neat, but it should not accentuate class differences. Among some cultures, it is considered rude to refuse food if it is offered. Extra effort to show acceptance and respect at the beginning of a relationship may help to win the trust of a family who is suspicious of outsiders.

Evaluation and Assessment

When completing an evaluation or assessment, the service provider must realize that most evaluation and assessment procedures have not been standardized for a variety of ethnic and socioeconomic groups and are therefore inappropriate to use with members of these groups. In addition, few instruments for infants and toddlers have been rigorously standardized, and even fewer are reliable or valid for culturally different populations. Many nonstandardized procedures may also be culturally biased. Anastasi (1988) stated that it is "futile to try to devise a test that is free from cultural differences. The present objective in cross-cultural testing is rather to construct tests that presuppose only experiences that are common to different cultures" (p. 357). Hughes (1992) warned that screening minority infants with tests standardized for Anglo-European, middle-class infants and interpreting differences as deficits may not be warranted: "It is recognized in child development literature that although major milestones are achieved by most infants throughout the world, the rate of development and the context of developmental expressions differ among cultures" (p. 171).

Walton and Nuttal (1992) provided considerations for evaluating preschoolers with diverse cultural backgrounds, which is also relevant for evaluating and assessing younger children. Anderson and Goldberg (1991) have compiled strategies to ensure that culturally competent practices are used in screening, evaluating, and assessing young children (see the Appendix at the end of this chapter).

Setting IFSP Outcomes

Cultural considerations are essential when determining child and family outcomes in the IFSP process (Paget, 1991; Thompson-Rangel, 1992). Family members' concerns, resources, priorities, desired outcomes, and preferred methods for achieving outcomes are filtered through their cultural perspectives. The service provider needs to incorporate practices that are consistent with and respectful of the family's culture in order to achieve intervention outcomes. Reaching consensus with family members on their IFSPs helps to ensure successful outcomes.

Family members are the ultimate decision makers on the IFSP team. The team must be sensitive to cultural, economic, or individual differences that affect a family's ability to negotiate complex systems. The service provider needs to understand a particular family's values and communication styles in order to provide family members with information that is useful to them in making decisions for the child. Conflicts can arise in any decision-making process. When the service provider and family view decisions from different cultural perspectives, the opportunity for conflicts increases. Gonzalez-Mena (1992) provided tips about allowing cultural conflicts to arise and responding in a sensitive, respectful manner.

SUMMARY

Diversity is a complex and often controversial issue. This chapter emphasizes the importance for those working in early intervention to explore their values, skills, and knowledge related to family diversity. The chapter suggests a way to begin a continuous process of rethinking methods for working with people who have diverse life experiences.

A framework and strategies for working toward cultural competence are proposed for service providers and programs. We assert that the ongoing process of working toward cultural competence is similar to that of working with diverse families in general. A four-step process is offered for strengthening cultural competence: 1) exploring one's own cultural attitudes, values, and practices; 2) understanding some of the sources of family diversity, such as culture, family structure, socioeconomic status, and parents who have disabilities; 3) understanding the barriers encountered by families in gaining access to and participating in early intervention; and 4) developing early intervention services that are responsive to diverse families.

Specific suggestions are given for guiding diverse families through the IFSP process. Service providers are encouraged to consider differences in communication styles and perspectives when building relationships with families. In addition, it is paramount to think about how diversity influences the evaluation and assessment of a child as well as the delineation of child and family outcomes in the IFSP process. Several modifications in procedures and approaches to accommodate differences based on cultural or other sources of diversity are discussed as well.

DISCUSSION QUESTIONS

◆ ◆ ◆

1. What is the importance of understanding your own cultural values when working in early intervention?

2. Four sources of family diversity are discussed in this chapter: cultural diversity, structural diversity, living in poverty, and parents with disabilities. It is also noted that some families face multiple challenges. Are there different ways in which to approach a family based on the kind of diversity they represent? If so, what are those ways? In what ways would approaching all families be the same?

3. How can the system in which you work be changed to help make it accessible to a range of families?

4. Is it important to have general information about different ethnic groups? Does such information lead to stereotyping families?

5. What should a person do if he or she disagrees with a family's decision about a child, a decision that is based on cultural values?

6. Suppose Sheila, the speech-language pathologist who is about to meet the Xiang family, had called you a week before meeting the Xiangs. What suggestions could you offer to help Sheila and her team develop a partnership with this family?   ◆

REFERENCES

Anastasi, A. (1988). *Psychological testing.* New York: Macmillan.

Anderson, M., & Goldberg, P. (1991). *Cultural competence in screening and assessment: Implications for services to young children with special needs ages birth through five.* Minneapolis, MN: PACER Center.

Anderson, P., & Schrag Fenichel, E. (1989). *Serving culturally diverse families of infants and toddlers with disabilities.* Washington, DC: National Center for Clinical Infant Programs.

Benn, R. (1993). Conceptualizing eligibility for early intervention services. In D.M. Bryant & M.A. Graham (Eds.), *Implementing early intervention: From research to effective practice* (pp. 18–45). New York: Guilford Press.

Brookins, G.K. (1993). Culture, ethnicity, and bicultural competence: Implications for children with chronic illness and disability. *Pediatrics, 91*(5), 1056–1062.

Bruder, M.B., Anderson, R., Schutz, G., & Caldera, M. (1991). Niños Especiales Program: A culturally sensitive early intervention model. *Journal of Early Intervention, 15*(3), 268–277.

Campt, D. (1992). Barriers to interventions with black clients. *Newsletter of the Clearinghouse for Drug Exposed Children, 3*(3), 1–3.

Carnegie Corporation Task Force on Meeting the Needs of Young Children. (1994). *Starting points: Meeting the needs of our youngest children.* New York: Author.

Chan, F., Lam, C.S., Wong, D., Leung, P., & Fang, X. (1988). Counseling Chinese Americans with disabilities. *Journal of Applied Rehabilitation Counseling, 19*(4), 21–25.

Chan, S. (1990). Early intervention with culturally diverse families of infants and toddlers with disabilities. *Infants and Young Children, 3*(2), 78–87.

Children's Defense Fund. (1993). Unsung heroes. *Children's Defense Fund Reports, 15*(1), 4.

Christensen, C.M. (1992). Multicultural competencies in early intervention: Training professionals for a pluralistic society. *Infants and Young Children, 4*(3), 49–63.

Christensen, C.P. (1989). Cross-cultural awareness development: A conceptual model. *Counselor Education and Supervision, 28,* 270–287.

Condeluci, A. (1991). *Interdependence: The route to community.* Orlando, FL: PMD Press.

Cross, T.L., Bazron, J.B., Dennis, K.W., & Isaacs, M.R. (1989). *Towards a culturally competent system of care: A monograph on effective services for minority children who are severely emotionally disturbed.* Washington, DC: Child and Adolescent Services System Program (CASSP) Technical Assistance Center.

Cunningham, K., Cunningham, K., & O'Connell, J.C. (1986). Impact of differing cultural perceptions on special education service delivery. *Rural Special Education Quarterly, 8*(1), 2–8.

Edmunds, P., Martinson, S., & Goldberg, P. (1990). *Demographics and cultural diversity in the 1990s: Implications for services to young children with special needs.* Chapel Hill, NC: National Early Childhood Technical Assistance System.

Einbinder, S.D. (1992). *A statistical profile of children living in poverty: Children under three and children under six, 1990.* Unpublished manuscript, Columbia University School of Public Health, National Center for Children in Poverty, New York.

Espe-Sherwindt, M., & Crable, S. (1993). Parents with mental retardation: Moving beyond the myths. *Topics in Early Childhood Special Education, 13*(2), 154–174.

Gonzalez-Mena, J. (1992). Taking a culturally sensitive approach in infant-toddler programs. *Infants and Young Children, 47*(2), 4–9.

Gray, D.B., & Schimmel, A.B. (1993). Future directions for research on reproductive issues for people with physical disabilities. In F.P. Haseltine, S.S. Cole, & D.B. Gray (Eds.), *Reproductive issues for persons with physical disabilities* (pp. 339–354). Baltimore: Paul H. Brookes Publishing Co.

Hanline, M.F., & Daley, S.E. (1992). Family coping strategies and strengths in Hispanic, African-American, and Caucasian families of young children. *Topics in Early Childhood Special Education, 12*(3), 351–366.

Hanson, M.J., & Lynch, E.W. (1992). Family diversity: Implications for policy and practice. *Topics in Early Childhood Special Education, 12*(3), 283–309.

Hanson, M., Lynch, E.W., & Wayman, K. (1990). Honoring the cultural diversity of families when getting data. *Topics in Early Childhood Special Education, 10*(1), 112–131.

Harry, B. (1992). Developing cultural self-awareness: The first step in values clarification for early interventionists. *Topics in Early Childhood Special Education, 12*(3), 333–350.

Hughes, S. (1992). Serving culturally diverse families of infants and toddlers with disabilities. *Infant-Toddler Intervention, 2*(3), 169–177.

Individuals with Disabilities Education Act. (1990). *The new Individuals with Disabilities Education Act (Senate Bill 1106, Section 6786): Special supplement to Education of the Handicapped (17*[5]). Alexandria, VA: Capitol Publications.

Individuals with Disabilities Education Act (IDEA) of 1990, PL 101-476. (October 30, 1990). Title 20, U.S.C. 1400 et seq: *U.S. Statutes at Large, 104,* 1103–1151.

Individuals with Disabilities Education Act Amendments of 1991, PL 102-119. (October 7, 1991). Title 20, U.S.C. 1400 et seq: *U.S. Statutes at Large, 105,* 587–608.

Kalyanpur, M., & Rao, S. (1991). Empowering low-income black families of handicapped children. *American Journal of Orthopsychiatry, 61*(4), 523–532.

Kanemoto, J.S. (1987). Cultural implications in treatment of Japanese American patients. *Occupational Therapy in Health Care, 4*(1), 115–125.

Kohls, L.R. (1984). *The values Americans live by.* Washington, DC: Meridian House International.

Krajewski-Jaime, E.R. (1991). Folk-healing among Mexican-American families as a consideration in the delivery of child welfare and child health care services. *Child Welfare, 70*(2), 157–167.

Leung, E.K. (1988, November). *Cultural and acculturational commonalities and diversities among Asian Americans: Identification and programming considerations.* Paper presented at the symposia of the Council for Exceptional Children and Ethnic and Multicultural Concerns, Dallas.

Locust, C.S. (1985). *American Indian beliefs concerning health and unwellness.* Tucson: University of Arizona, Native American Research and Training Center.

Lynch, E.W. (1992). Developing cross-cultural competence. In E.W. Lynch & M.J. Hanson (Eds.), *Developing cross-cultural competence: A guide for working with young children and their families* (pp. 35–59). Baltimore: Paul H. Brookes Publishing Co.

Lynch, E.W., & Bakley, S. (1989). Serving young children whose parents are mentally retarded. *Topics in Early Childhood Special Education, 12*(3), 26–38.

Lynch, E.W., & Hanson, M.J. (Eds.). (1992). *Developing cross-cultural competence: A guide for working with young children and their families.* Baltimore: Paul H. Brookes Publishing Co.

Lynch, E.W., & Hanson, M.J. (1993). Changing demographics: Implications for training in early intervention. *Infants and Young Children, 6*(1), 50–55.

Marshall, C.A., Martin, W.E., Thomason, T.C., & Johnson, M.J. (1991). Multiculturalism and rehabilitation counselor training: Recommendations for providing culturally appropriate counseling services to American Indians with disabilities. *Journal of Counseling & Development, 70,* 225–234.

Matsuda, M. (1989). Working with Asian parents: Some communication strategies. *Topics in Language Disorders, 9*(3), 45–53.

McCormack, G.L. (1987). Culture and communication in the treatment planning for occupational therapy with minority patients. *Occupational Therapy in Health Care, 4*(1), 17–36.

McCubbin, H.I., Thompson, E.A., Thompson, A.I., McCubbin, M.A., & Kaston, A.J. (1993). Culture, ethnicity, and the family: Critical factors in childhood chronic illness and disabilities. *Pediatrics, 91*(5), 1063–1070.

McGonigel, M.J., Johnson, B.H., & Kaufmann, R.K., (1991). *Guidelines and recommended practices for the individualized family service plan* (2nd ed.). Bethesda, MD: Association for the Care of Children's Health.

McKnight, J. (1995). Community: Will we know it when we see it? *Wingspread Journal, 17*(3), 8–9.

Morrow, R.D. (1987). Cultural differences—Be aware. *Academic Therapy, 23*(2), 143–149.

National Center for Children in Poverty. (1995). *Number of poor children under six increased from 5 to 6 million 1987–1992* (Vol. 5, No. 6). New York: Columbia University School of Public Health.

National Commission on Children. (1991). *Beyond rhetoric: A new American agenda for children and families.* Washington, DC: Author.

Orlansky, M., & Trapp, J.J. (1987). Working with Native American persons: Issues in facilitating communication and providing culturally relevant services. *Journal of Vision Impairment and Blindness, 81*(4), 151–155.

Paget, K.D. (1991). Early intervention and treatment acceptability: Multiple perspectives for improving service delivery in home settings. *Topics in Early Childhood Special Education, 11*(2), 1–17.

Patterson, J.M., & Blum, R.W. (1993). A conference on culture and chronic illness in childhood: Conference summary. *Pediatrics, 91*(5), 1025–1030.

Pinderhughes, E. (1988). *Understanding race, ethnicity, and power.* Elmsford, NY: Pergamon.

Ramer, L. (1992). *Culturally sensitive caregiving and childbearing families.* White Plains, NY: Education and Health Promotion Department, March of Dimes Birth Defects Foundation.

Roberts, R.N. (1990). *Workbook for developing culturally competent programs for families of children with special needs.* (2nd ed.). Washington, DC: Georgetown University Child Development Center and the Maternal and Child Health Bureau.

Rogler, L.H., Malgady, R.G., Costantino, G., & Blumenthal, R. (1987). What do culturally sensitive mental health services mean? *American Psychologist, 42*(6), 565–570.

Smart, J.F., & Smart, D.W. (1991). Acceptance of disability and the Mexican American culture. *Rehabilitation Counseling Bulletin, 34*(4), 357–367.

Thomason, T.C. (1991). Counseling Native Americans: An introduction for non-Native American counselors. *Journal of Counseling & Development, 69,* 321–327.

Thompson-Rangel, T. (1992). The Hispanic child and family: Developmental disabilities and occupational therapy intervention. *Developmental Disabilities Special Interest Newsletter, 15*(1), 2.

Toubbeh, J.I. (1985). Handicapping and disabling conditions in Native American populations. *American Rehabilitation, 11*(1), 3–10.

Turner, A. (1987). *Multicultural considerations. Working with families of developmentally disabled and high-risk children: The Black perspective.* Paper presented at the Infant Development Association Conference, Los Angeles. (ERIC Document Reproduction Service No. ED 285 360)

Vergara, E.R. (1992). Special issue on cultural diversity: From the guest editor. *Developmental Disabilities Special Interest Section Newsletter, 15*(1), 1.

Walton, J.R., & Nuttal, E.V. (1992). Preschool evaluation of culturally different children. In E.V. Nuttal, I. Romero, & J. Kalesnik (Eds.), *Assessing and screening preschoolers: Psychological and educational dimensions* (pp. 281–299). Boston: Allyn & Bacon.

Wayman, K., Lynch, E.W., & Hanson, M. (1990). Home-based early childhood services: Cultural sensitivity in a family systems approach. *Topics in Early Childhood Special Education, 10*(4), 56–75.

Westby, C.E. (1990). Ethnographic interviewing: Asking the right questions to the right people in the right ways. *Journal of Childhood Communication Disorders, 13*(1), 101–111.

Yacobacci-Tam, P. (1987). Interacting with the culturally different family. *Volta Review, 89*(5), 46–58.

Zuniga, M.E. (1992). Families with Latino roots. In E.W. Lynch & M.J. Hanson (Eds.), *Developing cross-cultural competence: A guide for working with young children and their families* (pp. 151–180). Baltimore: Paul H. Brookes Publishing Co.

Appendix

CULTURAL COMPETENCE IN SCREENING AND ASSESSMENT
Implications for Services to Young Children with Special Needs Ages Birth Through Five

◆◆◆

The following strategies were selected from the interviews we conducted, a review of literature, and the experiences of PACER and NEC*TAS staff. They are offered as suggestions for examining ways to ensure cultural competence in serving families from diverse backgrounds who have young children with disabilities or special needs. It is our hope that this section can serve as a tool for looking at and developing a personal framework that will ensure cultural competence in screening and assessment.

STRATEGIES FOR PART H AND 619 COORDINATORS AND OTHER POLICY MAKERS

1. Become knowledgeable about the cultural groups in your state, region, and local community when planning culturally sensitive screening and assessment policies, and deliver services that support the cultural uniqueness of the communities you serve.
2. Recruit people who have diverse cultural and linguistic backgrounds from state, regional, and local communities to serve on policy-making committees regarding the screening and assessment of young children with culturally and linguistically diverse backgrounds.
3. Develop a mission statement and implementation plan to address cultural competence issues in screening and assessment.

This appendix is reprinted by permission from Anderson, M., & Goldberg, P.F. (1991). *Cultural competence in screening and assessment: Implications for services to young children with special needs ages birth through five*. Minneapolis, MN: PACER (Parent Advocacy Coalition for Educational Rights) Center (4826 Chicago Avenue South, Minneapolis, MN 55417-1098; [612] 827-2966 **[V/TTY]**).

4. Develop communication networks and linkages with group leaders from ethnic and cultural minorities regarding cultural competencies in screening and assessment.

5. Develop "best practice" standards and guidelines for culturally competent screening and assessment.

6. Provide incentives for the recruitment and training of bilingual and bicultural personnel in early intervention services and screening and assessment.

7. Require staff training on cultural competence skills in screening and assessment, and set standards for professional cultural competence.

8. Find training and demonstration projects that utilize culturally competent standards in the screening and assessment process.

9. Create policies and systems that have cross-cultural screening and assessment philosophies and practices.

10. Recruit and retain people who have diverse cultural and linguistic backgrounds at all levels of involvement. Hire consultants to assist systems and agencies in the recruitment, training, and retention of people from a diversity of cultural/linguistic backgrounds.

STRATEGIES FOR PARENTS

1. Talk with other parents in your community for recommendations about schools, clinics, and providers they have used for screening and assessment.

2. Look for professionals and other providers who are familiar with and knowledgeable about your cultural and linguistic community and skilled in screening and assessing young children. Ask how experienced the provider is in screening and assessing children from your cultural group.

3. Become part of a network of other parents and professionals to gain support and information.

4. Insist that professionals and other providers be bilingual and bicultural or that skilled interpreters or mediators be used and that other staff receive ongoing training in cultural competence.

5. Look for cultural and linguistic sensitivity in the screening and assessment process. Are forms and information presented in your language? Is assistance available to help you fill out the forms, if needed? Is your child's screening and assessment being done in familiar settings using objects and routines other children in the community are exposed to?

6. Learn to trust your feelings and instincts about what does or does not work for your child and family.

7. Share cultural information that will assist professionals in understanding your child. For example, "My child is not walking yet be-

cause in my community children are often carried until age 2." You, as a parent and family member, know your child better than anyone else.

8. Communicate with professionals and other providers so that the screening and assessment process for your child and family is culturally sensitive and competent. Statements such as "I am not comfortable with my child being tested using those toys. He has never seen them before" or "Children in my community do not sit in chairs to do work at a table. Could he sit on the floor instead?" can help to make certain your child receives a nonbiased screening and assessment.

9. Know your rights regarding nondiscriminatory screening and assessment and other special education due process rights. Become involved with your local, community, and state advocacy groups.

10. Know where to turn for advocacy and assistance. If you think your child's screening and assessment has not been culturally sensitive, be sure to go to the agency and tell someone so that changes can be made.

STRATEGIES FOR PROFESSIONALS WORKING WITH FAMILIES FROM VARIOUS CULTURAL AND/OR LINGUISTIC GROUPS

1. Individualize the screening and assessment process for parents as well as for children. Children and other family members may be at various levels of acculturation and may require similar or varying degrees of modifications, adaptations, or support, such as language interpretation.

2. Do a self-assessment of your own cultural background, experiences, values, and biases. Examine how they may affect your interactions with people from other cultural groups.

3. Begin the screening and assessment process at the point the parents are. Find out their concerns, why they are coming to you, and what they hope you can provide.

4. Take the time to establish the trust needed to fully involve the family in the screening and assessment process.

5. Use bilingual and bicultural staff or mediators and translators, whenever needed. Try to maintain a consistency of providers to allow the family to establish an ongoing communication.

6. Allow for flexibility of the process and procedures. You may need to meet with parents at their job site or call them when they return home from their job. You may need to modify test items to ensure cultural competency.

7. Conduct observations and other procedures in environments familiar to the child. These may be at the home of the child's grandmother, outdoors, or at the parent's worksite.

8. Provide assistance and be flexible in establishing meetings with parents. This might include providing for child care of siblings, transportation to a meeting site, or meeting the family in their home.

9. Participate in staff training on cultural competence skills in screening and assessment. Strive to achieve standards for professional cultural competence.

10. Conduct ongoing discussions with practitioners, parents, policy makers, and members of the cultural communities you serve.

2

FAMILY SYSTEMS AND FAMILY-CENTERED CARE

Audrey L. Begun

◆◆◆

OBJECTIVES

◆◆◆ By completing this chapter, the reader will

- Become familiar with the concepts and terminology of family systems theory
- Learn the key elements of a family systems perspective
- Understand that families are dynamic, developing systems
- Learn to recognize some of the factors that influence the course of family development
- Become familiar with the concepts of family adaptation and adjustment
- Recognize inappropriate assumptions about families whose children have disabilities ◆

Since the mid-1970s, fields such as social work, nursing, psychology, education, medicine, and allied health have increasingly recognized the importance of working with families. To support an individual, a service provider must understand and work within the environment in which that person grows, develops, and functions. For nearly all young children, that context is the family. Although young children have experiences outside of their families, many of those experiences are selected, guided, and shaped by their families. The commitment to family-centered practices in early intervention was given new life by the passage of Part H of the Individuals with Disabilities Education Act (IDEA) of 1990, PL 101-476.

Family-centered care is sometimes misunderstood to mean simply working with parents to obtain assessment information or enlisting parents as supplementary professional providers of therapy. There are at least two problems with this interpretation. First, families often include not only parents but also sisters and brothers, aunts and uncles, cousins, grandparents, and pets. Some families include stepchildren, foster children, half brothers, half sisters, boyfriends, girlfriends, special friends, or neighbors. Second, to view parents as information sources or as providers of therapy is to miss completely the transforming power of the family-centered approach.

The implications of a family-centered perspective extend far beyond the need to think of additional roles for parents or to acknowledge that families include people other than parents. This is a relatively new way to view the relationships among child, family, and service provider—with the family at the center and the service provider as a collaborator. This deceptively simple statement has profound implications for early intervention practices. This chapter provides theoretical concepts and practical information in support of a family-centered perspective.

THE JOHNSON STORY

Tiffany was born 3½ years ago and is the first child of Dorothy and Earl Johnson. At 13 months of age, Tiffany was hospitalized for 6 weeks following an unexplained series of seizures. She was in a coma for 2 weeks. Before that time, there was nothing unusual about her development. Tiffany had been able to name several objects and people clearly and had been walking steadily on her own for a couple of months. "Until that night, she was just our own regular Tiffany, bouncing through each day," recalled Earl. Regarding the initial hospital period, Dorothy said,

> I died inside. I was screaming scared, but I had to hold it all together to deal with the doctors and the cast of thousands who got involved. All I could think was that she was lost to me forever. Even if she didn't die, who was she now? Where was the part of her that was *her*?

By the time Tiffany came home, she was able to lift herself on her hands and knees, but she could not move around in any kind of intentional way. She would occasionally produce some sounds in response to what was going on around her, but she could no longer form syllables or words. She played with familiar and favorite tabletop toys much as she always did. It seemed to the Johnsons that Tiffany had lost some coordination skills but that her thinking and problem-solving abilities had not changed. She still recognized her family: Dorothy, Earl, and the family dog, as well as the grandmother and aunt whom she saw frequently.

Dorothy said that her mother and older sister were "wonderful" through everything. They listened to her without judging or giving too much advice. They understood her and conveyed a belief that she has always been and still is a good mother. They also showed Dorothy and Earl that they still loved Tiffany and were eager to learn how to live with her since her hospitalization. Growing up, Dorothy had been close to an aunt who had mental retardation, and she had some contact with a cousin with severe learning disabilities. Both of these people were from her father's side of the family. (Dorothy's father had recently died.) Dorothy always admired her mother's authentic and practical manner of relating to these two in-law relatives. She also said that she can talk with her sister about the daily hassles and pleasures of child rearing the way any two mothers do. Her sister understands that although Tiffany's needs present her family with some unusual challenges, their lives are like those of other families with young children.

Earl's parents have responded quite differently. Their initial reaction was, "It didn't come from our side of the family." Earl and Dorothy were saddened but not angered or surprised. This response was in character for his parents. They do not handle crises well, and it is their nature to look for quick solutions. They persistently pursued information that might help to solve, cure, or fix Tiffany's problems. Earl's cousin by adoption began having tonic-clonic seizures when he and Earl were school-age boys. Earl's parents were accepting of this nephew, but they never discussed openly his seizure disorders.

When Tiffany was born, Earl's parents delighted in her every achievement. She was their first grandchild. Earl says that his parents never stopped loving Tiffany and that they still accept her, but they do not really seem to accept her differences. When she achieves something new (i.e., something that she had been able to do before her hospitalization or something that other children do at an earlier age), they become silent rather than excited. Earl pointed out, however, that they still pamper Tiffany as much as they did before and as much as they do their other grandchildren.

Dorothy and Earl have developed a child-centered household. A generous assortment of therapeutic toys and wheeled riders for Tiffany to "accidentally practice on" are scattered throughout the house. The family has regular visits with a neurologist, a neuropsychologist, a pediatrician, a physical and occupational therapy team, and a speech-language therapist, as well as with various nursing, social work, and clinical staffs. One of Earl's greatest frustrations in retrospect, and, delights, was the doctors' initial pessimism: "They said she would absolutely never talk and would probably never walk. She'd need a wheelchair and would never go to college. How could they have been so sure? Look how wrong they've been!"

A few months before Tiffany's third birthday, her baby sister Tonya arrived. Five months later, Tiffany began attending an early childhood program at the nearby public school 5 mornings each week. Within a few months, Tiffany clearly was able to say her own name, "Moose" (i.e., the dog's name), "Like it," "No more," and "Down." Around the same time, she first let go of the wheeled toys and began to walk on her own. According to Earl, she was "wobbly, and with odd, rubbery joint movements, but walking!"

The Johnsons are considering child care or nursery school options for Tiffany's afternoons. She loves her early childhood class, but it offers her little opportunity to make friends with children without disabilities, something that is important to Earl and Dorothy. Dorothy even thinks that she might be ready to return to the dental hygiene career that she interrupted when Tiffany was first hospitalized.

Dorothy and Earl agree that, much of the time, they do not really think about Tiffany's needs as different or special. They are just a part of her. As Dorothy said,

> Everyone thought I was grieving the "perfect life" my daughter should have had. I was really grieving the fact that I couldn't stop this terrible thing from happening to my baby. I was powerless to protect her from the hurt. And I was afraid of my own vulnerability.

At times of transition, however, special issues do arise. For example, their choice of nursery schools will depend to a great extent on teachers' willingness both to learn how Tiffany communicates and to view her as a typical 3-year-old who happens to have special needs. Dorothy also said,

> When she has a seizure now, I get a kind of quietly desperate fear. Not about the seizures or anything, but about the foreverness and the helplessness. And I have a private worry about the mixed-blessing days when Tonya will overtake her sister, doing things that Tiffany can't. Well, I'll face that when I come to it, won't I? I won't have any choice.

THEORETICAL BASIS FOR FAMILY-CENTERED CARE

To work effectively with a variety of families whose young children have special needs, service providers need to understand concepts developed by those who study families. Furthermore, family members can become more effective in directing their own lives if they are aware of the forces and processes operating in their own families.

This chapter is organized around three basic conceptual constructs: 1) *family systems,* 2) *family development*, and 3) *family adaptation and adjustment*. These concepts can be applied to families with various structures, histories, or ethnic and cultural backgrounds. They can be applied to all families, not just those whose children have disabilities. These constructs can help people working in early intervention to understand families who have young children with disabilities.

Family Systems Perspective

The family is not simply a collection of individuals but a complex system. To understand a family, it is not enough to know who the members are. The experience of living in a family involves the emotional bonds and interaction patterns that exist among family members. It also includes the family's history, values, goals, dreams, and belief systems. Finally, it involves interactions outside the family.

Key Concepts

To engage in family-centered care, it is important to adopt a family systems perspective.There are five concepts basic to a family systems perspective:

1. The family as a system is more than the sum of its parts.
2. Change in one part of the family affects the entire family system.
3. Subsystems are embedded within the larger family system.
4. The family system exists within a larger social and environmental context.
5. Families are multigenerational.

Taken together, these concepts imply that within families there are members who interact as interdependent parts of a larger network. These concepts further imply that the family system itself is an integral part of other social systems. Finally, they imply that the family system is dynamic and characterized by change.

Exploration of Key Concepts

The Family as a System Is More than the Sum of Its Parts Families develop their own sets of rules, dynamics, patterns, boundaries, behaviors, strategies, and procedures, all of which are directed toward maintaining the system. The family as a whole has substance, meaning, and form; a family has a life beyond the members' individual lives. Family members share what is termed a *joint identity* (Broderick, 1993, p. 188). Preservation of the family system becomes a major goal of the family and all of its members. Sometimes members work toward this goal even when it is contrary to what might be in their own personal best interests. For example, as adults, brothers and sisters of people with developmental disabilities sometimes maintain weighty responsibilities for their families by continuing to help meet the emotional and instrumental needs of their siblings and parents, despite their own personal, individualized life goals.

Like any other living system, a family system is composed of interdependent members whose interactions create patterns of relating that do not exist with any single facet of the system. One important implication of this interdependence among family members lies in what Minuchin (1974) termed the *circularity of influence* between individuals and their social environments. Although we are used to thinking about the ways in which an individual's environment affects that individual's behavior and development, it is important to consider the impact of that individual on the environment as well. For example, although it is clear that parents' behaviors affect children's development, the ways in which children shape their parents' behaviors are often ignored. A person with developmental disabilities is affected profoundly by his or her family environment, but that person also has a profound impact upon the family system. This circular pattern of influence—a person affects others who affect that person who affects others and so on—can be found in any family relationship that exists over time.

Circularity of influence implies that no simple cause-and-effect explanation describes sufficiently what is observed in a family's behavior. For example, if the parents of a child with autistic behavior seem to hold back from engaging the child actively, it does not necessarily follow that their restraint caused the child's social reserve. It is equally likely that the parents' restraint developed over time in response to the child's subtle social cues and responses to their earlier attempts at social engagement. The family's pattern of interaction may have evolved as a result of a circular pattern of influence, child-to-parent and parent-to-child, over many interchanges over time.

Change in One Part of the Family Affects the Entire Family System
Because of the interdependence that exists among members of a family system, changes experienced with regard to any facet of the system will cause changes for the system as a whole. The term *family generalization* has been applied to this principle for situations in which interventions directed toward improving parent–child interactions have extended benefits to other relationships in the family (Baker, 1989; Griest & Forehand, 1982). Sometimes these are direct, primary benefits. For example, when a child who has been cared for exclusively by the mother begins school, life changes dramatically for the mother as well as the child. Similarly, when a person with mental retardation develops a chronic or serious medical condition, life changes not only for that person but also for each caregiver and support system member—especially parents and siblings.

Sometimes the effects on other family members are less direct. For example, as a child develops language skills, there are dramatic changes in the way in which family members and others in the child's social environment interact with that child; they begin to relate differently. (This is a direct effect of a developmental change in an individual.) This change in the child, however, also changes the way in which other family members are able to interact with each other. For instance, they may have to modify what they talk about or how they talk. There may not be conversational space either for them to talk to one another when the new speaker is around or for the new speaker to express ideas. This is an indirect effect of changes in the child on the rest of the family system.

This aspect of family systems has considerable import for early intervention service providers because interventions with a child reverberate throughout a family system. For example, a suggested change in the feeding routine of an infant with special feeding needs may result in more pleasant mealtimes for the whole family, more energy by parents for each other and for all of the children, and better feelings toward the infant by siblings. A change in how a parent handles a child's behavior problems may affect not only the child's behavior but also the parent–child relationship as well as their interactions with other family members. Medications to control a child's hyperactivity may result in changes not only in the child and in the child's relationships with parents, brothers, and sisters but also in how and how much the parents and siblings are able to interact with one another. These sorts of changes may be either positive or negative, or both. The point is that changes in one part of the system, whether in an individual or in a relationship, will affect the entire system. The changes may be profound or subtle, but they have systemwide ramifications that are not confined to a single individual or relationship.

Subsystems Are Embedded within the Larger Family System   It would be awkward and cumbersome for family members if they always acted and interacted as a whole group. Instead, various members often have specialized patterns of interaction that do not include other members directly. For example, the intimate partners in the marital subsystem may be more effective than the family as a whole in managing the budget or making decisions about household tasks. In a two-parent family of five people, the parent–child subsystem becomes apparent whenever the mother and father operate together as a unit in relation to the three children.

Traditionally, professionals consider three common family subsystems:

1. The marital subsystem—intimate partners (e.g., husband and wife)
2. The parental subsystem—parent and child[1]
3. The sibling subsystem—brothers and sisters

This, however, is not an exhaustive list. At times, other subsystems, such as those including grandparents or other members of the extended family, may be engaged. Diverse subsystems emerge in families with ex-spouses, step or half relations, foster children, and/or many siblings or siblings of widely spaced ages. Within a family, there are multiple, overlapping, and changing subsystems. For instance, "The development of the parental subsystem may overshadow, at times, the spousal system in the early child-rearing years. With a chronically ill child in the forefront, the spousal subsystem may disappear or be frustrated to a dangerous degree" (Rosman, 1988, p. 299).

Subsystems are not independent of the larger family system. Their character may mimic or defy the values, norms, beliefs, and patterns of the family system. Either way, subsystems are influenced by the larger system. They provide opportunities for family members to interact as individuals. The dynamics of subsystems may be considerably more sensitive to the individuality of family members than is the system as a whole.

The Family System Exists within a Larger Social and Environmental Context   The family system should be viewed as being embedded within a broader social context. Families do not exist in isolation, independent of their environments. They exist as systems that nest in and interact with

---

[1]Family systems experts disagree about how to define the parental subsystem. Both the parent–child and parent–parent subsystems are important components of most families.

other social systems. According to the social-environmental view of individual development, which was strongly influenced by Bronfenbrenner (1979), a person develops within a *microsystem* of social interactions that occur within a context of increasingly remote rings of other systems. An analogous pattern of nested system rings can be developed for the family.

The family's most immediate ring—the family's *microcosm*—includes neighbors, extended family members, friends, children's peers, co-workers, and others who shape the day-to-day experiences of family living. This realm of the family's ecological context is sometimes referred to as the family's informal support system.

The neighborhood, broader community, and formal service systems form a family's *mesocosm*—the middle-range context of the family's exchanges. These systems have a somewhat more indirect—but no less profound—impact on the family's daily living. These other systems might also include the following: formal service delivery systems, the school system, parents' workplaces, and systems that help define a family's culture and ethnicity (e.g., church, clubs, social organizations). Interactions at this level tend to be more formalized and regulated and are characterized less by interactions between individuals. This facet of the family's ecosystem is generally referred to as the formal system of supports.

Family life is profoundly affected by a host of somewhat more remote systems: mass media, government, and economic and political events. This *macrocosm* of societal, cultural, and historical systems provides a broad and sweeping (yet often intangible) influence on family living. Although the effects of this outermost ring are as significant as those of the more intimate inner rings, the effects of the former are often more difficult to identify, and tend to be buffered, screened, and modified before they are actually felt by family members. Societal trends, norms, values, events, and belief systems that affect socialization and social life for individuals and families are involved. Race relations, regional demographic changes, social reform movements, economic recessions and "boom" periods, and involvement of the nation in war are some examples of the influences of the macrocosm. For families of children with disabilities, societal attitudes of particular importance include those regarding mothers who work; fathers' involvement in child rearing; the impact of the Americans with Disabilities Act (ADA) of 1990, PL 101-336; professional accountability; health care reform; and the costs and quality of special education services.

An important implication related to Bronfenbrenner's (1979) main point about the ecosystem is that in order to change an individual, it is often appropriate, and necessary, to make changes in that individual's environment. By extension, to provide family-centered care, it may be more effective to support a family from outside the family system than to try to change the system directly. For example, working with the news media (i.e., macrocosm) to publicize more consistently the triumphs and positive contributions of people with developmental disabilities may have a powerful impact on a family's feelings about life with a child who has disabilities. As another example, respite care services (i.e., meso-cosm) may improve parents' relationships with their babies. For some families, this may be preferable to providing family therapy (i.e., micro-cosm) or special parenting classes.

A final implication of a family ecosystem is tied to the circular nature of influences in systems. Although family contexts have an impact on families, families also have an impact on their contexts. Family members can effect changes in formal service delivery systems, policies, and societal norms, as well as in their personal support systems and in the delivery of services (Bradley, 1992). One can utilize a family Eco Map (Hartman, 1978) to depict a family's social context and the nature of interactions between the family and their surrounding systems. Figure 2.1 shows a family Eco Map (or family portrait) for the Johnson family.

Families Are Multigenerational   At any point in time, observers of a family system get only a single "snapshot" view. Family members, how-ever, are keenly aware of their family's history and future. Although a household may include only two generations (i.e., parents and children), the family system is affected by much more. Members of other genera-tions do not have to be present or even alive to influence a family's life. It is not unusual for families to have four or more generations that are im-portant in their lives. Most family systems overlap with a number of other family systems from the past, present, and future. A family genogram is often utilized to help map the generational patterns and re-lationships in a family system (Hartman, 1978; McGoldrick & Gerson, 1989).

ACTIVITY: *Appointment Observation*

◆ ◆ ◆   After obtaining the consent of everyone involved, join a family for a visit to another service provider or agency. Observe what goes on as the fam-ily interacts within this larger social context. Think about all the interac-tions between family members and agency personnel (including interac-tions that occur for reasons other than scheduled appointments) from the family members' points of view. What can be learned from this expe-rience about interactions with families?   ◆

The Johnson Family and the Family Systems Perspective

The Johnson family story reflects a number of the key concepts basic to the family systems perspective. Families have characteristics all their

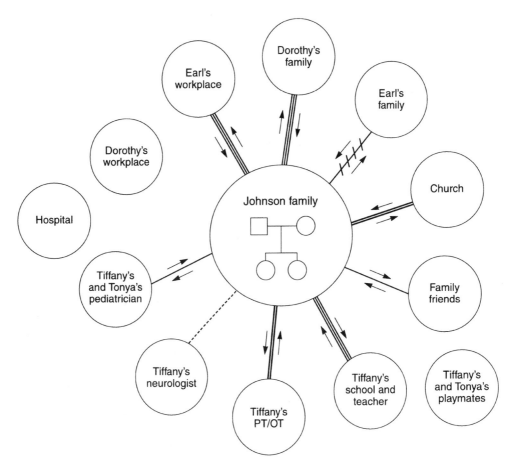

Figure 2.1.   Family Eco Map illustrating the family system within a social context.

own, and preservation of the Johnson family's characteristics is important to the parents. They see their family, including Tiffany, as regular
people with some unusual needs. In meeting those needs, they look for
ways to affirm their similarities to other families. They express a powerful sense of awareness of their past, present, and future existence, and
family members have powerful influences on each other. Tiffany's
growth allows Dorothy to consider returning to work. The attitudes and
behaviors of Tiffany's aunt and grandmother have an effect upon the
mother's behavior. Just by her presence, Tiffany's younger sister Tonya
redefines many of Tiffany's interactions with Dorothy and Earl.
Tiffany's steady progress reinforces Earl's optimism, and he in turn encourages her ongoing development. This family operates as a system
that is more than the sum of its parts. Circular patterns of influence
exist as well.

The most obvious effect of Tiffany's medical crisis has been on her own development and capabilities. Clearly, however, these effects have influenced other family members and the family system as a whole. Dorothy quit her job, which resulted in a loss of income. The family subsequently entered into a world of professionals and specialists in the disability field, forcing Earl and Dorothy to assume new roles and to undergo considerable self-education regarding Tiffany's disabilities. Routines have been altered, as necessitated by Tiffany's care needs and by frequent visits with service providers. The changes experienced by Tiffany have affected the entire family system. In the future, as Dorothy returns to work, Tiffany enters school, and Tonya matures, each of these changes will again affect the family system.

The Johnson family includes a marital subsystem (i.e., Dorothy and Earl as a couple), sibling subsystems (i.e., Tiffany and Tonya, Dorothy and her sister), and a parental subsystem (i.e., Dorothy and Earl interacting as parents with their children). Additional significant subsystems include the following: the grandparents with their grandchildren, Dorothy with her mother, Dorothy and Earl with his parents, and perhaps family members with the dog. These subsystems operate within a broader family context of values, beliefs, and relationships expressed by the general family system.

The Johnson family's most intimate social environment includes extended family and friends. These people provide considerable amounts of emotional and instrumental support. Tiffany's therapists, the service delivery system in the family's state and community, Earl's workplace, and child care resources constitute a secondary ring of interactions. Doctors' negative predictions may have induced Tiffany's parents to work harder on her behalf, and therapists' suggestions may have influenced the Johnsons's decisions about toy purchases, family routines, room arrangements, and so forth. The media, the status of research and knowledge about Tiffany's disabilities, and societal attitudes toward disabilities constitute the Johnsons' outermost ring of interactions. All have an impact on the Johnsons' day-to-day existence. This family system exists within and interacts with a larger social and environmental context.

Finally, the Johnson family is definitely multigenerational in nature. Earl's and Dorothy's parents are important parts of their lives. At the same time, Earl's and Dorothy's childhood experiences with people with disabilities affect their current values and their parenting of Tiffany. Tiffany and Tonya have an impact upon the grandparents as well.

Recognizing the Language and Behavior of a Family Systems Perspective

Professionals vary in the extent to which they have adopted a family systems perspective. Their words and actions provide clues, as shown in Table 2.1.

Table 2.1. Recognizing the family systems perspective

Nonsystems	Systems
The service provider:	The service provider:
Thinks of a family as a household or grouping of people.	Asks about the household members, extended family, multiple generations, neighbors, and others important to the family.
Considers how a planned intervention will affect the child.	Considers how a planned intervention will affect the child and other members of the family and their relationships with one another.
Makes assumptions about a person's role in the family based on position in the family (e.g., parent, only child, twin, youngest).	Asks questions about a person's interactions with various family members, recognizing that individual roles develop as a result of many interactions over time.
Focuses on the here and now in assessment and planning for intervention.	Takes account of the family's views of their own past, present, and future in assessments and intervention planning with the here and now as part of a long-range continuum.
Considers the welfare and development of the child with disabilities and teaches other family members how to support that child's growth.	Considers the welfare and development of the child with disabilities and teaches other family members how to support that child's growth while also looking for ways to support the growth and development of other family members and the family system as a whole.
Gives credit (or assigns blame) to family members for a child's progress (or problems).	Considers factors outside the family as well as the family's own actions and attitudes when exploring needs or discussing progress with the family.

Family Development Perspective

Families are dynamic and characterized by change. One important way in which change occurs in families relates to their development over time. Over time, and in response to developmental pressures, families alter and modify their functions. For example, a family's functions evolve as an infant becomes a toddler, a preschooler, a school-age child, and eventually an adolescent and young adult. Some of the areas in which their functions shift involve attachment behaviors, caregiving, discipline, and communication. Remember, however, that the child is not the only family member in the system who is developing. Parents, siblings, and extended family members continue to develop throughout their lives as well.

Models of Family Development

Over time, family systems respond to a combination of the following four common triggers for developmental change:

1. Developmental change in a single member
2. Change in one of the subsystems or relationships between or among family members
3. Change in family membership due to birth, adoption, death, marriage, separation, "launching" a young adult, reentry of a launched member, and so forth
4. Pressure for change from the family's ecological context in the form of changing resources or changing social expectations, demands, or norms

These forces can act singly or in combination to promote developmental change in families. For example, when a young child reaches an age at which community norms concerning school entry and greater independence from the family are triggered, the school system places new demands on the family and imposes expectations about the child's relationships with other family members. During this common occurrence and with no changes in family membership, three forces for family development are engaged: 1) developmental change in a single member (i.e., the child), 2) change in one of the subsystems or relationships between or among family members (i.e., new tasks for the parent–child subsystem), and 3) pressure for change from the family's ecological context (i.e., the community's expectation that the child will attend school).

Several different family development stage models have been presented since the 1940s. (For descriptions of some of these theories, see Aldous [1990] or Duvall [1977].) Most of these theories identify a series of stages or *developmental crises* that generally confront families. In each stage, the family attempts to resolve the challenges and issues particular to that stage and achieve a stable plateau after a specific transition. Developmental challenges and issues, regardless of the stage during which they occur, require change on the family's part. Mobilizing for change is stressful and renders the family more vulnerable for a time.

The stages (five in some models and as many as 28 in others) generally involve such life events as

- Becoming a couple
- The birth of a first child
- Raising children and launching the first child
- Concluding child rearing by launching the last child
- Facing the end of life

Unfortunately, these models generally fail to predict development in the diverse range of families in U.S. society. Many families in the late 20th century do not follow such normative patterns. Some families, such as those raising children outside of marriage, undergo certain stages in a different order. Others, such as those comprising couples who do not have children, skip some stages altogether. Reconstructed families—families with children from prior marriages and perhaps from the current marriage as well—can experience more than one stage at a time. Some families' cultural norms regarding the pace and timing of developmental events are different from those of the majority of families in the United States. Indeed, "A rigid application of psychological ideas to the 'normal' life cycle can have a detrimental effect if it promotes anxious self-scrutiny that raises fears that deviating from the norms is pathological" (Carter & McGoldrick, 1989, p. 4).

Along these lines, it is useful to view families of children with disabilities as following a course of development that is affected, but not arrested, by their experiences. They should be viewed as different, not deficient, in nature. For example, a child's disability may alter the form and timing of family launching, but launching is not necessarily precluded. Furthermore, this child's family may be in a state of *décalage*—representing multiple phases of development simultaneously—rather than operating fully within a single stage at any given time. For example, the family of a young child with multiple disabilities may continue to face demands usually associated with the early stages of development (e.g., diapering, transporting, feeding) while simultaneously facing the more typical demands of the school years, such as school and peer involvement.

> The parents of a child [with a developmental disability] are meeting a challenge at once heroic and ordinary. The heroism, though unsought, is undisputed. Who would voluntarily change places? Yet most daily challenges for these parents and children are pretty much the same ordinary ones that occupy all families. (Baker, 1989, p. vii)

Clearly, stage models are generally insufficient to explain the experiences of families of children with special needs. Additional information about family change is needed. It is helpful to consider a *life events model* that is superimposed over the stages of family development.

Paranormative Family Events

It should be noted that all change (e.g., happy events, sad events, anticipated and unanticipated events, marriages, births, retirements) is stressful for families. Many families experience changes that are considered in U.S. society to be out of the ordinary. These are termed *paranormative family events*. Paranormative family events are those that do not generally happen to a majority of families. The birth of a baby with developmental disabilities or exceptional health care needs is an example of a paranormative event. The baby's family experiences all of the normative activities associated with having a new family member, yet simultaneously experiences the paranormative challenges involved with meeting the baby's special needs. Adoption as a means of bringing a new member into the family is another example of a paranormative family event.

Off-time events are those that occur either much earlier or much later than usual for a given culture. They represent one type of paranormative family event. Families of children with disabilities frequently experience off-time events. For instance, they must relate to schools (or school-like places) long before children ordinarily enter kindergarten. They share with others (e.g., therapists, special education teachers, medical personnel, psychologists) the responsibilities of nurturing and caregiving in ways that most families do not. And the child's achievement of personal milestones, such as walking, talking, or potty training, may occur years later than is typical.

As mentioned previously, any transition from one stage of family development to another, whether the catalyst for the transition is normative and predictable or paranormative and unanticipated, can produce stress for a family system. A family does not, however, face this stress in a vacuum. Families experience the catalyst in the context of their past developmental experiences and their own unique character, including established interactional patterns, past crises (and their resolutions), myths and secrets, cultural norms and taboos, and the legacies of past generations.

Past experiences, norms, values, beliefs, culture, and ethnicity affect a family's interpretation of events. If the issues and themes of current developmental events intersect with those of past events, even a minor current stressor may have overwhelming consequences for a family. Another family facing a similar event but without relevant past events may experience relatively little stress. A family's developmental history has a profound impact on their response to current developmental events (Carter & McGoldrick, 1989). For example, although two babies may be born with similar disabilities and their families may be given identical information about their conditions, the families' responses will probably be quite different despite the similar circumstances. The impact of a family's past experiences is one reason for these disparate responses.

Families do not usually anticipate paranormative events, and therefore are often unprepared for them. Because these events are relatively uncommon, the support and resource systems of a community may be inadequate to meet a family's needs. Thus, paranormative events have a great potential to disrupt a family's developmental course. Experiencing a paranormative event does not mean that a family is no longer typical. However, paranormative events do heighten the potential for crisis because the family and its support systems may lack the resources and experiences necessary to adapt to new situations. Normative family tasks such as supporting children's development among peers, planning for their futures, and launching them into the adult world often have paranormative aspects for families of children with disabilities.

Initial Diagnosis What are some of the paranormative developmental issues that frequently confront individuals with developmental disabilities and their families? The first and perhaps most recognizable issue involves a child's initial diagnosis. For some families, it is evident at the time of or soon after birth that an infant has significant developmental differences and special needs. For others, there are prolonged periods of tension during which they suspect that the infant or young child has "something wrong," but they are unable to confirm their suspicions with a formal diagnosis.

In both situations, the family experiences a crisis period. The crisis involves recognizing that their lives have been changed forever—that they are now operating outside a predictable flow of family life. In the second situation, in which the family experiences a prolonged period of doubt before diagnosis, the actual diagnosis may be a relief rather than a crisis in itself. They have already been living with their suspicions yet trying to live as though there were no problems.

The initial crisis phase can be a critical time for professional intervention. A family in crisis has a powerful need for honest, factual, relevant information. The family is often desperately seeking all sorts of information about the child's disabilities: what to expect in the near and distant future, what services and treatments are available, who in the professional community is recommended to work with these problems and with families, how other families have adapted, and so forth. A family also may have a need for supportive services that reinforce or strengthen members' adaptation skills. For some families, this may be the first serious crisis that members weather together. They may not be confident in their abilities to cope with crisis. Other families may have experienced prior crises but without gaining the skills and resources that result in competency and coping skills. At any rate, families in this phase should be respected as families in transition. What they exhibit and express is crisis behavior, not long-term resolutions.

Coming to Terms   A second issue faced by families of children with disabilities is that of coming to terms with the ways in which their lives are changing. Many parents and service providers describe a period of intense grief experienced by family members following the recognition or diagnosis of a child's disabilities. Kübler-Ross's (1970) developmental theory of grieving losses is often applied in such situations. A family's behavior may comprise an erratic progression (with a lot of backsliding) through the stages of denial, anger, bargaining, and acceptance. Developmental models suggest that resolution of this grief will follow a cyclical, fluctuating course rather than a smooth, sequential pattern (Seligman & Darling, 1989).

As a family continues to develop, a renewed sense of distress may be triggered by changes in the member with disabilities (e.g., the discovery of additional problems). In addition, Birenbaum (1971) indicated that missed or delayed developmental milestones act as triggers for renewed grief in the family. Families also may experience a sense of dissonance between societal norms regarding family life and their own experiences.

This dissonance is often associated with a reactivation of sadness and grief. It is important to note, however, that families whose children have disabilities do not exist in a permanent state of grieving, but periodically revisit it.

Discovering the Service Delivery System A third paranormative issue experienced by families of children with disabilities is that of having to engage a complex service delivery system, arranging support services for the child and perhaps for other family members. Families vary in the degree to which they find it difficult to request help. Boundaries, values and norms, past experiences, and specific needs affect families' skills and comfort in using community resources. Few parents are prepared to serve "executive parent" functions (Keniston & The Carnegie Council on Children, 1977); that is, they have been socialized to care for their children, not to be recruiters, hirers and firers, advocates, consumers, coordinators, or professionals. Becoming a participant in the service delivery system is a unique developmental task for some parents, just as it is for the child with disabilities. This challenge forces many families to confront and to articulate their positions about previously unexamined values (e.g., specialized schooling versus integration or inclusion, family living versus out-of-home placement). It also may foster intimacies with people outside of the family that seem somewhat artificial. Professionals intrude upon very personal, intimate aspects of family life, no matter how delicately and respectfully they collaborate.

Relations with Outside World A fourth challenging issue involves a family's relations with extended family members and the outside world. Family members may experience dramatic shifts in the balance and nature of their microlevel support systems. Many find that their energies are necessarily redirected so that they cannot support the friendships and casual relationships they once experienced. Others find there are few people outside of the family who can understand their situation and appreciate the child with special needs. Not all families become limited by such an "inward spiral." Many create ties to a community of families whose children also have special needs.

The Johnson Family and the Family Development Perspective

The Johnson family system is dynamic and changes over time. There have been multiple triggers for development. Tiffany's illness and the developmental achievements of both Tiffany and Tonya represent some individual changes that prompted changes in the family system. The Johnsons's marriage, Tiffany's and Tonya's births, and the death of Dorothy's father all triggered development associated with membership changes. As Tiffany and Tonya continue to develop, the outside world will place expectations upon the Johnsons to enroll the girls in school, prepare them for independence, and rework their attachment relationships.

The Johnsons have progressed through several normative family development stages and have completed the transitions to couplehood and parenthood. They are now entrenched in the child-rearing stage. In the future, they will face issues regarding the launchings of Tiffany and Tonya, retirement, and living as older adults. The extended family has also experienced a host of normative developmental stages: Earl and Dorothy were launched into adulthood, their parents became grandparents, and several of the aunts and uncles have become parents.

In addition to these normative events, the Johnsons are also continuing to respond to the paranormative event of Tiffany's disabilities. At first, Earl and Dorothy experienced her illness and sudden loss of skills as a crisis that required the activation of their adaptive energies to restore a sense of balance. Earl and Dorothy have resolved their initial grief, but, like many families adapting to an unending situation, they reexperience feelings of sadness and vulnerability periodically. Tiffany's disabilities also have led to a much greater involvement with the medical, social services, and education systems than is experienced by most families. Seeking child care, a normative task, has paranormative implications because Tiffany's special needs must be considered.

The Johnsons' experience of Tiffany's disabilities was influenced by more than the event of Tiffany's diagnosis. It was the result of interactions among some of the family's past experiences, values, and beliefs. There were preexisting implications of having a family member with a disability. And one part of the extended family system (i.e., Earl's parents) has always had difficulty in handling events that do not lend themselves to quick fixes or cures.

Recognizing a Family Development Perspective

Service providers vary regarding the extent to which they have adopted a developmental view of families. Table 2.2 suggests some ways to recognize a family development perspective.

ACTIVITY: *Support Group Meeting*

◆ ◆ ◆   Attend a family support group meeting. Check ahead of time to be sure you will be welcome at the meeting. Place yourself in the "audience" role, not in that of a participating service provider. With everyone's consent, listen to what family members have to say about their lives. How does the family developmental perspective facilitate your understanding of what family members are saying?   ◆

Table 2.2.   Recognizing the family development perspective

Nondevelopmental	Developmental
The service provider:	The service provider:
Relies on a clear, "snapshot" view of the family at one point in time; thinks that the way a family appears now is the way they have always been and always will be.	Regularly seeks new information for an updated, "video" view of the family, recognizing that families are dynamic and evolve over time.
Thinks about each event as a distinct, discrete factor in a family's life.	Thinks about the interaction of past, present, and future events for the family.
Considers how a paranormative event may affect a family.	Looks at a paranormative event within the context of normative life cycle events for the family.
Views an event as either normative or paranormative.	Distinguishes between the normative and paranormative aspects of an event, rather than classifying an entire event as normative or paranormative.
Looks for a cause for some aspect of a family's behavior.	Is aware of multiple forces acting on a family and rejects simple cause-and-effect explanations of family behavior.
Thinks of family development as a linear, steplike pattern (i.e., "onward and upward").	Recognizes the nonlinear nature of family development and appreciates the stops, starts, and cyclical patterns.

Family Adaptation and Adjustment Perspective

Clearly, families whose children have disabilities vary tremendously with regard to their adjustment and adaptation. Some families face the challenges of raising a child with disabilities with a great deal of grace and a sense of competence, without seeming to be hurt by the experience. They make comfortable adjustments and continue to be healthy families. There are other families for whom the presence of a child with disabilities is overwhelming; many of these families simply endure the experience. Some families are overwhelmed or were struggling prior to the appearance of their children's disabilities, and the extra demands have a relatively small impact on their lives, or, conversely, a catastrophic impact. The challenges associated with rearing children with disabilities can enable some families to develop close, strong bonds of affection. In short, there is tremendous diversity and heterogeneity among families of children with disabilities.

In the past, much of the literature examined the hazards associated with having a family member with disabilities (Lavigne & Ryan, 1979; San Martino & Newman, 1974). A host of potential problems for family members were identified. These problems were explained by such "emotional morbidity" factors as guilt, disproportionate sharing of attention and other resources, and excessive child care demands. Although these explanations were sometimes helpful in understanding families with problems, they did not apply to all families of children with disabilities. This section examines the reasons that families vary so dramatically in their responses to having children with disabilities.

Resilience

The concept of resilience is derived from the field of public health epidemiology. It is based upon the observation that an entire population can be exposed equally to something harmful, yet many do not succumb to its effects. This is an important concept to keep in mind when assessing the impact of a child's disabilities upon the family system. A family's resilience does not depend only on the nature of the crisis they face. A family meets the crisis in a condition of relative strength or weakness, and their social and physical environment affects responses to the crisis as well. The concepts of vulnerability and risk help to explain the broader issue of resilience among family systems (Begun, 1993).

Vulnerability   Vulnerability encompasses all that families bring to the situations and challenges they encounter. Factors such as family dynamics (i.e., communication styles, cohesion, roles, relationships), values and belief systems, past experiences, and internal resources (e.g., finances, energies, special skills or knowledge) tend to make a family more or less vulnerable. Vulnerability is also affected by a family's adaptability and responses to stressful events. Some families are relatively rigid and do not respond well to stressful events. Others are appropriately flexible and adapt quite readily. Still others are relatively chaotic and find it difficult to organize their responses. For a particular situation, a family can be seen as being somewhere on a continuum that spans the range from high vulnerability to low vulnerability and that comprises all of these characteristics.

Risk   Risk reflects the environmental context and external resources of families. The level of risk can be increased or diminished by the presence or absence of societal pressures, neighborhood and community factors, historical trends, formal support services, positive role models, resources, and informal support systems. Families can be seen as being anywhere on a continuum that spans the range from high to low levels of environmental risk and that comprises all of the environmental characteristics just discussed.

Figure 2.2 can be used as a gross index of family resilience. It shows the intersection of the two dimensions of vulnerability and risk that results in four levels of probability that a problem will develop.

Levels of Resilience   Resilience is greatest among families for whom vulnerability and risk are low. Such families do not need preventive interventions and may require only the maintenance of those factors that account for their low vulnerability and low risk. The level of resilience is lowest and the probability of difficulties is highest among families for whom both vulnerability and risk are high.

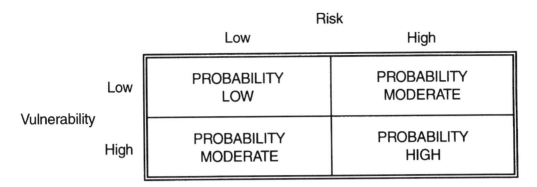

Figure 2.2.   Probability of a problem.

Imagine a family living in poverty with no health insurance and a history of alcoholism in both parents. These factors contribute to high vulnerability. The same family also experiences conflicts in relationships with friends, neighbors, and/or extended family members and lives in a "service poor" community where economic conditions are volatile. These factors contribute to high risk. This family has a high probability for serious problems when responding to an event such as the discovery of a child's disability. Preventive interventions for families such as this should be designed 1) to reduce vulnerability or increase resistance to stressors, and 2) to decrease environmental risks or add protective factors from outside the family system.

Moderate resilience is experienced by families who are low in one dimension and high in the other. For such families, effective prevention and intervention strategies should be geared toward decreasing the vulnerability or risk factors and building protective factors that keep them out of the low probability/high resilience group while at the same time maintaining the factors that keep them out of the high probability/low resilience group. Knowing about vulnerability and risk can help service providers to avoid common, unjustified assumptions about certain kinds of families and their resilience (or lack thereof). For example, it is not safe to assume that a single-parent family with a child with disabilities has a high probability for developing problems. The family *may* be vulnerable as a result of limited resources. They *may* be socially isolated and therefore at risk. At the same time, they *may* be a family entrenched in a supportive network of extended family that provides for the family's emotional and instrumental needs. Neither vulnerability nor risk stems directly from the parent's being single.

Similarly, living in poverty does not necessarily mean that a family has a high probability for problems. Indeed, poverty is often associated with a host of conditions (e.g., poor health, limited access to health care, limited education, substandard housing, discrimination in service delivery practices, unsafe neighborhoods) that make families vulnerable or that may place them at risk. Because a particular family living in poverty may or may not experience these conditions, however, it cannot simply be assumed that the probability for difficulty is high. Poverty alone does not preclude resilience. Furthermore, an inability to move a family out of poverty does not imply an inability to effectively intervene to prevent or reduce the probability of adjustment difficulties for that family.

Finally, consider a middle-class family in which both parents live together in a home located in a safe, stable community. This family's level of resilience if one of their children has disabilities cannot be assumed. The family's values may stress high academic and athletic achievement. Family members may believe that they should be self-sufficient and therefore may find it difficult to accept help. Perhaps one of the adults has a sibling who was institutionalized as a child. Perhaps one or both parents depends upon alcohol or other substances as a means of coping with difficulties. The family may have very limited experience in adapting to unanticipated changes, and the environment, although safe, may not be completely supportive. The school district may focus on college-bound students to the detriment of others. Perhaps their friends and neighbors look down on those who use publicly funded services such as early intervention. These possibilities have important implications for intervention planning. It is essential to address the actual risk factors (e.g., lack of resources, need for respite care and other supportive services). It is not helpful just to identify needs as the results of poverty or single parenthood—facts that intervention cannot change. Furthermore, it is essential to address the factors that support families and foster resilience in order to work with families from a "strengths perspective" (Saleebey, 1992).

Adaptation and Adjustment Processes

Adaptation refers to the processes that help a family 1) to achieve a comfortable balance, and 2) to promote the growth and development of individual members and the system as a whole. Adaptation involves changes in the system that evolve over relatively long periods of time and have long-term consequences. It includes changes in a family's roles, rules, patterns of interaction, perceptions, and norms. *Adjustment*, by contrast, is a relatively short-term response, usually to a specific event or stressor. Adaptation and adjustment are affected by the nature of a stressful event, the family's resources, and their perceptions of the event.

As noted previously, families whose children have very similar disabilities often respond quite differently. One way of examining the reasons that families might differ in their responses to life events is offered in the *ABC–X* and the *Double ABC–X* family crisis models (Cowan, 1991; McCubbin, Cauble, & Patterson, 1982; Seligman & Darling, 1989). Basically, there exists an interaction among the specific demands of a new situation (A), a family's resources for dealing with the situation (B), and the family's definition or perceptions of the event (C). The interaction results in the crisis itself (X). *Doubling* includes not only the challenges inherent in the A event, but also the existence of any other, separate situations that may occur as well as the family's successes or failures in attempting to cope (the Double A component). It also includes (as the Double B component) the resources that were previously available to the family as well as the coping resources that strengthened or developed as a result of responding to the event. The Double C component refers to the family's redefinitions of the situation along with their perceptions of and the meanings they attach to the event. The Double *ABC–X* model reflects the dynamic, evolving nature of the adjustment, adaptation, and coping processes.

For two families facing the identification of an infant's disabilities, the actual stressful events are similar. Therefore, different responses may be caused by differences in resources or perceptions. Perhaps one family has a strong support system, adequate health care, and access to information when they want it. The other family may find it more difficult to adjust and adapt to their new circumstances because they lack these resources. Perhaps one family believes that God sends children with disabilities to families who have extra love, whereas the other family believes that their child's disability represents a punishment from God.

The two families' adjustment and adaptation also will be affected by their different perceptions of the similar events. It would be an oversimplification to assume that differences in the families' responses are simply related to differences in the degrees of severity of their children's disabilities. It is important to keep in mind not only the nature of the children's disabilities but the families' resources and perceptions about their children as well. Furthermore, it is important to remember that these three domains (as well as the crisis itself) continue to change and evolve as the families cope over time.

Support Systems A concept that is repeated throughout this chapter is that of family support systems. Support systems are critical elements of the adjustment and adaptation processes. They represent the people and other systems that provide input (i.e., nurturing, information, resources, energy, services) into the family system. Several issues related to family support systems should be examined; one way to conceptualize a family's support system is through the Eco Map (Hartman, 1978; see also Figure 2.1).

Costs and Benefits Although a family's support systems are largely responsible for input into the family system, there are also costs to the family for establishing and maintaining support systems. Some costs, or outputs, can be financial if the family pays to obtain certain services or information. But costs can take other forms as well. A friend may be happy to listen to a frustrated or depressed family member and may expect a turn to talk at a later time. A neighbor may babysit in exchange for getting free grass cutting. Support from a church or synagogue depends to some extent on the family's participation in a religious community. It has also been suggested that some programs distort parents' rights to be involved in providing services to their children by placing excessive demands and expectations for involvement upon them (Baker, 1989; Turnbull & Turnbull, 1982).

Most families are able to find a satisfactory balance between the benefits and costs of their support system. They "get as good as they give." They find satisfaction, self-esteem, and an outlet for creative energies by giving support to others and ensuring that their own needs are well met. Some families, however, find it difficult to achieve a satisfactory balance between themselves and their support systems. There may be gaps in the types of supports available or certain supports may not be available in sufficient quantities. In addition, the energies that families expend to maintain support systems may be overwhelming, particularly if individuals outside the families are experiencing stressful life events themselves.

"Goodness of Fit"   It is vital for support systems to respond to families' unique concerns. Some families find it distressing that support systems seem to exist but do not respond to their individualized needs. Sometimes support systems misunderstand families' needs. Sometimes they give what is available regardless of whether or not it is needed. Some parts of support systems may have eligibility criteria that a family or child does not meet. For example, in some communities, respite care is available for families whose children have developmental disabilities, but not for families whose children have emotional disabilities. When there is a good fit between a family and support systems, the family's needs are satisfied and there is a comfortable balance between the family and support systems. Unfortunately, some families experience a less-than-optimal fit with support systems.

Formal and Informal Supports   Families vary in their use of formal, paid support services from professionals and agencies. Some families depend almost entirely upon such formal sources of support. Families also vary in their reliance on the informal support of relatives, friends, neighbors, and peers. Some families have rich, diverse informal support systems; others have little informal support available to them. Some families use substantial amounts of formal and informal support, whereas others use little of either kind of support. "Support groups composed of parents of [children and adults with disabilities] serve a number of functions, including (1) alleviating loneliness and isolation, (2) providing information, (3) providing role models, and (4) providing a basis for comparison" (Seligman & Darling, 1989, p. 44).

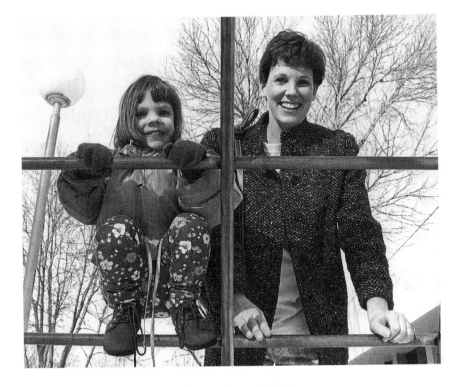

The Johnson Family and Adaptation and Adjustment

The family adaptation and adjustment perspective provides additional ways in which to view the Johnson family. The Johnsons seem to have adequate financial resources. Their communication and decision-making skills are functional. They have some relevant past experiences upon which to draw. There do not seem to be many other stresses acting upon the family, and they do not seem to be overwhelmed by difficulties. Dorothy and Earl have adequate parenting skills, and the family is appropriately cohesive and adaptable. For all of these reasons, the family's level of vulnerability is probably low, despite the vulnerability caused by Tiffany's disabilities.

The Johnsons' environment is not one of high risk. Adequate services are available and accessible, their social support system is functional, and there is no indication of any threatening or troubled interaction with the community (e.g., legal difficulties, police involvement, violence and crime hazards). Because the Johnsons are low vulnerability and low risk, they are similar to other low probability families in that they are probably resilient enough to resist most serious adjustment problems caused by Tiffany's disabilities. The probability of adjustment problems is low unless the family's circumstances change and they become more vulnerable or face greater risk.

The Johnsons' adaptation and adjustment have been influenced by the nature of Tiffany's disabilities, which began as a medical crisis and then developed into a long-term situation. Because Tiffany was a toddler when the crisis occurred, her parents were able to face several challenging transitions one at a time. They became parents first; they later became parents of a child with disabilities. They had the advantage of experiencing life as confident, competent parents. Many of Tiffany's needs have become somewhat predictable. Her seizures are not predictable, however, and they do therefore present additional adaptive challenges.

The family's resources are another influence on adaptation and adjustment. The Johnsons' resources—economic, physical, emotional, and interpersonal—have so far been adequate. By responding to Tiffany's situation for 2 years, they have developed new means to gather information, skills, and confidence. Their adaptation and adjustment are further affected by their perceptions of events. The Johnson family seems to view Tiffany's disabilities as presenting a series of challenges to be overcome, but not as overwhelming or devastating problems. They do not view themselves as deficient in comparison to other families (or in comparison to what they were before the discovery of Tiffany's disabilities). Rather, they view themselves as having some differences. This interpretation of events is supportive of positive adaptation.

The Johnsons seem to have found a satisfactory balance in their support systems. This may change, however, with the new demands resulting from Dorothy's return to work. The Johnsons have engaged a variety of supports that are both formal and informal in nature. Despite the fact that there have been and will continue to be periodic frustrations with elements of their support systems (e.g., Earl's parents, pessimistic doctors), these systems are generally meeting the needs of the family system quite effectively.

Recognizing an Adaptation and Adjustment View of Families

Service providers vary regarding the extent to which they are aware of adaptation and adjustment in families. Table 2.3 presents some points of comparison.

ACTIVITY: *Home Visits*

◆ ◆ ◆

Schedule a series of home visits with several families of young children with disabilities (with the consent of all involved, of course). These families should not be service recipients with whom you work. You are observing them as a student of family life, not in the capacity of a service provider. Before your visit

- Develop a tentative list of questions that will teach you about the family system, the family's development, and the family's adaptation.

- Think about the aspects of family interaction that you want to observe. What will they tell you about the system, development, and adaptation?

After your visit, write yourself a report that includes your questions and how you got (or did not get) them answered. Think about how you might restructure your approach to reports you write for your job so that they include information about systems, development, and adaptation. ◆

SUMMARY

This chapter presents a number of concepts related to adopting a family systems perspective in early intervention practice. These include discussion of the way that the system affects, and is affected by, its membership, as well as the multigenerational nature of family systems. It also includes issues related to change and the dynamic nature of family

Table 2.3.   Recognizing the adaptation and adjustment perspective

Nonadaptation	Adaptation
The service provider:	The service provider:
Makes general assumptions about how families are affected by their children's disabilities.	Acknowledges the tremendous variability among families' responses to their children's disabilities.
Assumes that resources are equally distributed across and within communities and that all families have equal access to those resources.	Recognizes the idiosyncratic nature of a family's resources.
Looks at the nature of the event when considering how it might affect a family.	Looks at the family's unique characteristics, event interpretation, and resources, as well as the nature of the event, when considering how an event might affect a family.
Believes that all families share common beliefs and values about disabilities, seeking help, and raising children (and/or that they share the beliefs of the service provider).	Recognizes that each family has their own beliefs and values that are based on past experiences, cultural backgrounds, and religion.
Refers to families' support systems as though every family has one, as though they are all similar, and as though they are always helpful.	Acknowledges the variability in family support systems as well as the costs and benefits of interacting with support systems.
Does not distinguish between formal and informal sources of support.	Is aware of the differences between formal and informal sources of support.
Thinks of adaptation as an immediate response to a challenge.	Distinguishes among adjustment, short-term responses, and adaptation that occurs gradually over a period of time.

systems, as well as how the family system interfaces with other systems in its ecological context. A developmental perspective is also applied to family systems, including a presentation of adaptation and adjustment issues related to normative and paranormative family life events. Vulnerability, risk, resilience, and protective factors are also discussed with regard to factors that affect family adaptation and adjustment processes.

DISCUSSION QUESTIONS

◆ ◆ ◆

1. What practices are employed that support the family as a system? What recommended practices for an individual child might interfere with the family as a whole? Discuss ways to expand upon the first group of practices as well as ways to modify recommended practices to better meet the needs of the family system.

2a. In what ways might a family with a child with disabilities develop subsystem dynamics that are different from those of other families? Why? In what ways are the differences adaptive? In what ways are they problematic? How do service providers potentially help or hinder this process?

2b. Discuss the development of subsystems in the Johnson family. In particular, develop your ideas about the experiences over time of Earl and Dorothy as a couple, of Earl and Dorothy as parents, and of Tiffany and Tonya as sisters.

3a. Identify ways in which young children "train" their parents regarding parenting roles. How else do children shape their social contexts (e.g., the child who stops crying when he or she is picked up and spoken to in a soothing voice is reinforcing this behavior and making the caregiver feel successful and competent; the caregiver is simultaneously reinforcing the child's cries for attention)? Then discuss ways in which this *behavioral dialogue* process can be affected by a child's disabilities.

3b. Parents who have reared other children competently may have to modify some of their skills and approaches in order to respond to a child with disabilities. What is the same about raising this child? What may seem to be different because of the child's unique traits? What is truly different? What if the Johnsons' second child were to develop disabilities similar to Tiffany's? How would family adjustment and adaptation be affected?

4. The following statements reflect a difference of opinion about the roles of parents in early intervention:

The time spent with a child by service providers can have a relatively small impact on the child's development. The impact of intervention can be greatly enhanced when parents extend treatment time by teaching the child to generalize new skills in settings beyond treatment sessions. Parents should be encouraged to take on this role, especially during the critically important early years.

Young children need their parents to be parents, not teachers or therapists. Encouraging parents to interact with their children in nonparental ways alters the family system in undesirable ways. Instead of professionalizing parents, we should support them in acquiring whatever information, support, or skills they need to function as effectively as possible in their roles are parents.

Where do you stand on the continuum of opinions on this issue? How might the family systems, family development, or adaptation and adjustment perspectives help to resolve these two points of view?

5. How do the "normal" family processes appear in the family of a young child with disabilities? For example, how might attachment and bonding still occur but appear different? How do we recognize what may look so different or be so subtle? ◆

REFERENCES

Aldous, J. (1990). Family development and the life course: Two perspectives on family change. *Journal of Marriage and the Family, 52*, 571–583.

Americans with Disabilities Act (ADA) of 1990, PL 101-336. (July 26, 1990). Title 42, U.S.C. 12101 et seq: *U.S. Statutes at Large, 104*, 327–378.

Baker, B.L. (1989). Parent training and developmental disabilities. *Monographs of the American Association on Mental Retardation, 13.*

Begun, A.L. (1993). Human behavior and the social environment: The vulnerability, risk, and resilience model. *Journal of Social Work Education, 29*(1), 26–35.

Birenbaum, A. (1971). The mentally retarded child in the home and the family life cycle. *Journal of Health and Social Behavior, 12*, 55–65.

Bradley, V.J. (1992). Overview of the family support movement. In V.J. Bradley, J. Knoll, & J.M. Agosta (Eds.), *Emerging issues in family support* (pp. 1–8). Washington, DC: American Association on Mental Retardation Monographs, No. 18.

Broderick, C.B. (1993). *Understanding family process: Basics of family systems theory.* Beverly Hills: Sage Publications.

Bronfenbrenner, U. (1979). *The ecology of human development.* Cambridge, MA: Harvard University Press.

Carter, B., & McGoldrick, M. (1989). Overview: The changing family life cycle— A framework for family therapy. In B. Carter & M. McGoldrick (Eds.), *The changing family life cycle: A framework for family therapy* (2nd ed., pp. 3–28). New York: Gardner Press.

Cowan, P.A. (1991). Individual and family life transitions: A proposal for a new definition. In P.A. Cowan & M. Hetherington (Eds.), *Family transitions* (pp. 3–30). Hillsdale, NJ: Lawrence Erlbaum Associates.

Duvall, E. (1977). *Marriage and family development* (5th ed.). Philadelphia: J.B. Lippincott.

Griest, D.L., & Forehand, R. (1982). How can I get any parent training done with all these other problems going on?: The role of family variables in child behavior therapy. *Child and Family Behavior Therapy, 4*, 73–80.

Hartman, A. (1978). Diagrammatic assessment of family relationships. *Social Casework, 59*(8), 465–476.

Individuals with Disabilities Education Act (IDEA) of 1990, PL 101-476. (October 30, 1990). Title 20, U.S.C. 1400 et seq: *U.S. Statutes at Large, 104*, 1103–1151.

Keniston, K., & The Carnegie Council on Children. (1977). *All our children: The American family under pressure.* San Diego: Harcourt Brace Jovanovich.

Kübler-Ross, E. (1970). *On death and dying.* New York: Macmillan.

Lavigne, J.V., & Ryan, M. (1979). Psychological adjustment of siblings of children with chronic illness. *Pediatrics, 63*(4), 616–627.

McCubbin, H.I., Cauble, A.E., & Patterson, J.M. (Eds.). (1982). *Family stress, coping, and social support.* Springfield, IL: Charles C Thomas.

McGoldrick, M., & Gerson, R. (1989). Genograms and the family life cycle. In B. Carter & M. McGoldrick (Eds.), *The changing family life cycle: A framework for family therapy* (pp. 164–189). Newton, MA: Allyn & Bacon.

Minuchin, S. (1974). *Families and family therapy.* Cambridge, MA: Harvard University Press.

Rosman, B.L. (1988). Family development and the impact of a child's chronic illness. In C.J. Falicov (Ed.), *Family transitions: Continuity and change over the life cycle* (pp. 293–309). New York: Guilford Press.

Saleebey, D. (1992). *The strengths perspective in social work practice.* New York: Longman.

San Martino, M., & Newman, M. (1974). Siblings of retarded children: A population at risk. *Child Psychiatry and Human Development, 4*(3), 168–177.

Seligman, M., & Darling, R.B. (1989). *Ordinary families, special children: A systems approach to childhood disability.* New York: Guilford Press.

Turnbull, A.P., & Turnbull, H.R. (1982). Parent involvement in the education of handicapped children. A critique. *Mental Retardation, 20,* 115–122.

RECOMMENDED READINGS

Baker, B.L. (1989). *Parent training and developmental disabilities.* Washington, DC: American Association on Mental Retardation Monographs,13.

Crnic, K.A., Friedrich, W.N., & Greenberg, M.T. (1983). Adaptation of families with mentally retarded children: A model of stress, coping, and family ecology. *American Journal of Mental Deficiency, 88,* 125–138.

Dunst, C., Trivette, C., & Deal, A. (1988). *Enabling and empowering families: Principles and guidelines for practice.* Cambridge, MA: Brookline.

Fewell, R., & Vadasy, P.F. (1986). *Families of handicapped children.* Austin, TX: PRO-ED.

Friedrich, W.N., & Friedrich, W.L. (1981). Psychosocial assets of parents of handicapped and nonhandicapped children. *American Journal on Mental Retardation, 85,* 551–553.

Gardner, A., Lipsky, D.K., & Turnbull, A.P. (1991). *Supporting families with a child with a disability: An international outlook.* Baltimore: Paul H. Brookes Publishing Co.

Healy, A., Keesee, P.D., & Smith, B.S. (1989). *Early services for children with special needs: Transactions for family support* (2nd ed.). Baltimore: Paul H. Brookes Publishing Co.

Kazak, A.E., & Marvin, R.S. (1984). Differences, difficulties, and adaptation: Stress and social networks in families with a handicapped child. *Family Relations, 33,* 67–77.

Lobato, D. (1983). Siblings of handicapped children: A review. *Journal of Autism and Developmental Disorders, 13,* 347–364.

Schilling, R.F., Gilchrist, L.D., & Schinke, S.P. (1984). Coping and social support in families of developmentally disabled children. *Family Relations, 33,* 47–54.

Shelton, T.L., Jeppson, E.S., & Johnson, B.H. (1987). *Family-centered care for children with special needs.* Bethesda, MD: Association for the Care of Children's Health.

Sloman, L., & Konstantareas, M.M. (1990). Why families of children with biological deficits require a systems approach. *Family Process, 29,* 417–429.

Stoneman, Z., & Berman, P.W. (Eds.). (1993). *The effects of mental retardation, disability, and illness on sibling relationships: Research issues and challenges.* Baltimore: Paul H. Brookes Publishing Co.

Turnbull, A.P., & Turnbull, H.R. (1986). *Families, professionals, and exceptionality: A special partnership.* Columbus, OH: Charles E. Merrill.

Unger, D.G., & Powell, D.R. (1980). Supporting families under stress: The role of social networks. *Family Relations, 29,* 566–574.

3

Parent and Service Provider Partnerships in Early Intervention

Peggy Rosin

◆◆◆

OBJECTIVES

◆◆◆   By completing this chapter, the reader will

- Know what is meant by the term *partnership*
- Know why a partnership should occur
- Understand how partnerships are developed and enhanced   ◆

> Striving to employ partnerships between parents and professionals as a way of influencing parenting competencies and effecting positive changes in children's behavior and development necessitates a major change in the typical role relationships between professionals and parents. Such a shift requires abdication of paternalistic approaches to helping relationships and adoption of empowerment, participatory involvement, and competency enhancement approaches to help-giving. (Dunst, Trivette, & Johanson, 1994, p. 211)

It is clear that with the advent of family-centered early intervention, there is a need to change how parents and providers view each other's roles in the process. How does one define the alliance between parents and service providers? The concept of *partnership* is receiving widespread attention in early intervention literature as a way to envision the emerging relationship between parents and service providers.

There is some concern that if partnership becomes a buzzword in the 1990s, it may lose its meaning and potential effectiveness (Kagan, 1991; Paget & Chapman, 1992). What is meant by partnership in the context of early intervention? The search for clear definitions of partnership has yielded multiple interpretations and some confusion. Goodman's (1994) perspective is that through empowerment and partnership, service providers relinquish their professional roles as information givers and simply defer to parents' requests. This interpretation of parent–professional partnerships seems extreme, cautious, and wrong. Goodman and many service providers are, however, struggling with the concept of partnership and how it affects their roles and boundaries when working with families.

With the emphasis on family-centered services, many service providers need to reexamine their roles in working with families. A not-too-old philosophical tradition saw professionals as experts who were primarily responsible for making decisions related to the services provided to children. Current practices in early intervention encourage service providers to give information and offer support in a manner that empowers parents. Confusion exists about what the relationship between parents and service providers should entail. This chapter explores several questions regarding partnerships between parents or caregivers and service providers in early intervention. Although it explores partnerships on a personal, person-to-person basis, other chapters in this book address equally important issues related to developing and nurturing partnerships through teams and with agencies (see Chapters 6 and 7, respectively).

GERMAINE JACKSON AND THE GLEASON FAMILY: STARTING OVER

Germaine Jackson has been a teacher with the Central City birth-to-3 program for about 9 months. Before she was hired, Germaine was an early childhood teacher for 8 years in a school district in a small town about 60 miles north of the city.

Germaine's mother lives in Central City and has recently had serious health problems. Because Germaine wanted to be close to her mother to help her out and give her two children the chance to see their grandmother more often, they recently relocated to an old neighborhood in Central City.

Germaine was shocked to see how the neighborhood had changed since she lived there about 10 years ago. She had earned her degree at the university in Central City and had raised her two children alone working various minimum wage jobs. Because she wanted a fresh start after she graduated, she moved to Shelby and accepted her job as an early childhood teacher.

Being part of the birth-to-3 home-based program is new for Germaine. She has already seen more than she can believe. She wonders how children grow up in such environments. It is not just the poverty (she grew up poor), but it seems to her that parents just don't care about their children the way they should. She sees parents make choices with which she does not agree. For example, the mother of one of the children in her caseload, Trisha Gleason, never seems to have diapers but always has cigarettes.

Today Germaine went to see Trisha Gleason and her infant son, Anthony, for her weekly visit. When Germaine arrived, Trisha as usual seemed surprised to see her despite the fact that they have met at the same time for 3 months. Frequently when Germaine arrives there is no answer at the door, so today she was glad to find that Trisha was at home. As Germaine entered, she noticed that Trisha was clearly agitated and seemed a little frightened. Germaine heard Anthony crying and screaming from down the hall. They both approached Anthony, and Trisha picked him up and comforted him. Anthony is typically a happy baby, so Germaine asked if there was something wrong. Trisha said, "No, he's just crabby because he didn't have no nap."

Trisha never seems to Germaine to be forthcoming, and she always seems to be holding back. Trisha often just nods or gives minimal responses when Germaine asks questions about Anthony or what is happening in their lives. As Germaine watches Trisha with Anthony, it brings back a flood of memories about her own two children and how hard it was raising them alone. It is clear to Germaine that Trisha adores Anthony even if she makes what Germaine thinks are bad choices.

As Trisha soothed and rocked Anthony, Germaine commented on the challenges she faced in raising her own children and talked about how hard it was to do. She commended Trisha's ability to quiet Anthony. Trisha asked Germaine a few questions about her children, and soon Trisha was really talking about her fears for Anthony and herself: how she was afraid that someone would take her child, how she was frightened by Anthony's father who sometimes came over drunk or doped up and started pushing her around, how Anthony was the best thing that ever happened to her, and how everyone talks about Anthony's problems and delays.

Germaine realized that Trisha was really talking to her, but she was not sure what to do with the information. When she was a classroom teacher, she spoke mostly to parents during conferences or through notes. Germaine was not sure what had happened, but it seemed as if she, Trisha, and Anthony had reached a new beginning.

WHAT IS MEANT BY PARTNERSHIP?

The concept of partnership can have different meanings for different people. The *American Heritage Desk Dictionary* defines the term *partner* as "One who cooperates with another in a venture, occupation, or challenge" (1981, p. 691). Dunst and Paget (1991) reviewed and integrated existing literature on parent–professional relationships and found no operational definition of partnership. Dunst et al. (1994) viewed partnerships as a major dimension of their model of empowerment. In this model, partnership refers to activities that are characterized by "interpersonal transactions." Paget and Chapman (1992) stressed that partnerships with parents constitute an ongoing process of problem solving. Critical to their definition of partnership as a process are the following: 1) partners learn to communicate and relate effectively, and 2) the structure and procedures of an early intervention program promote partnerships overtly (e.g., offering options to parents about their levels of involvement, asking about parents' preferences about scheduling and locations).

ACTIVITY: *Partnerships*

◆ ◆ ◆   Think of a relationship that you have had with someone that you thought was a partnership. What elements of that partnership did you value most? List three elements and briefly describe why you chose them. ◆

Although partnership may have no clear definition, there are elements common to all partnerships. People may not be able to say what a partnership is, but they know it when they see it. Vosler-Hunter (1989) identified a number of elements of partnership and collaboration, including the following: 1) mutual respect for skill and knowledge, 2) honest and clear communication, 3) open and two-way sharing of information, 4) mutually agreed-upon goals, and 5) shared planning and decision making. Dunst and Paget (1991) proposed a similar list of elements of partnerships that includes 1) mutual contributions and agreed-upon roles; 2) a desire to work together in pursuit of agreed-upon goals; 3) shared responsibility in taking action to achieve goals; 4) loyalty, trust, and honesty; 5) full disclosure of pertinent information between or among partners; and 6) parents in the roles of decision makers. Both sets of elements highlight parent–professional partnerships as reciprocal and mutual.

In Germaine's and Trisha's story, there seemed to be a turning point in their relationship. Some of the elements of partnership just described may be emerging in their relationship. For example, Germaine acknowledged Trisha's competence in comforting her son and affirmed her skills and knowledge as a parent. This is important in light of Trisha's fear that people may take her son from her. Perhaps Trisha's previous conversations with professionals were deficit oriented, building Trisha's sense of her lack of control with her son. Germaine also reflected on her own life and opened the door for a discussion about the challenges she faced. There was a mutual sharing of experiences.

Dunst et al. (1994) surveyed a group comprising parents and service providers and confirmed what were previously thought to be the essential features of partnerships. The 26 features listed most frequently on the survey were grouped into four categories: beliefs, attitudes, communicative styles, and behavioral actions. The definitions of these categories and the major characteristics associated with each are listed in Table 3.1.

In defining partnership, it is important to examine the four common misconceptions about parent–professional relationships discussed by Pletcher and Deal (1993). The first misconception is that partnership is synonymous with friendship. Although the concepts are similar in some ways, there are notable differences. For example, in a partnership, there is agreement on the purpose and the desired outcomes of the relationship, as specified in the individualized family service plan (IFSP). This is not necessarily the case in a friendship.

A second misconception is that a partnership entails an equal division of responsibility. Partnerships are dynamic, the relationship between or among partners changing over time and being dictated by the tasks at hand, circumstances, and resources. Coservice coordination describes the process by which a parent agrees that there can be negotiation about 1) who will assume service coordination duties, and 2) how the intensity of participation and the types of activities will vary (see Chapter 8). Although there is a partnership in coservice coordination, the relationship does not necessarily involve equal sharing as much as negotiation about who will do which tasks.

A third misconception about parent–professional partnerships is that only the goals and concerns of parents are addressed. In actuality, the sharing of information is bidirectional. Service providers have an obligation to supply parents with relevant, accurate, and up-to-date information to assist them in making informed decisions about their children and

Table 3.1.   Categories, definitions, and characteristics of partnerships

Category	Definition	Characteristics
Beliefs	Cognitive attributions about how one should act or ought to behave toward other people	Trust, mutual respect, honesty, acceptance, mutually supportive, nonjudgmental, presumed capabilities
Attitudes	Particular (emotional) feelings about a person, situation, or relationship	Caring, understanding, commitment, empathy, positive stance, humor, confidence
Communicative styles	Methods and approaches for information sharing between partners	Open communication, active listening, openness, understanding, full disclosure of information, information sharing
Behavioral actions	Behaviors that reflect translation of attitudes and beliefs into actions	Mutual respect, openness, flexibility, understanding, shared responsibility, mutual support, reciprocity, mutual agreement about goals, dependability, equality, humor, problem solving

From Dunst, C.J., Trivette, C.M., & Johanson, C. (1994). Parent–professional collaboration and partnerships. In C.J. Dunst, C.M. Trivette, & A.G. Deal (Eds.), *Supporting and strengthening families: Vol. 1. Methods, strategies, and practices* (pp. 197–211). Cambridge, MA: Brookline Books; reprinted by permission.

the outcomes of their IFSPs. Parents, in turn, offer their knowledge of their children and families and contribute to the information base used in making decisions.

The final misconception, discussed by Pletcher and Deal (1993), is that building partnerships takes too much time. Partnerships are not events; they are processes that happen over time as providers work together with families to develop and implement IFSPs. It is the way in which parents and service providers work together that makes a partnership. Achieving a partnership between or among people is an individual occurrence. How quickly or easily it happens depends on the characteristics of those involved. For some relationships, a partnership may never be achieved.

WHY SHOULD A PARTNERSHIP OCCUR?

A rationale for parent–professional partnerships can be developed using a variety of information, including the following: legal information, theoretical data, empirical data, and practical knowledge (Paget & Chapman, 1992; Salisbury, 1992). Building partnerships in early intervention is a win–win situation. All involved in a partnership can benefit, including the child.

Germaine's initial attitudes and judgments about Trisha's choices for Anthony and herself may have interfered with her ability to determine what Trisha actually thought and felt. This lack of communication between them could have had negative repercussions throughout the entire IFSP process. If an IFSP is developed after a partnership is established, it will be responsive to the family's concerns, priorities, and resources, and it will respect the family's cultural context as well.

At least three assumptions that stress the concept of partnership are related to the IFSP process: 1) families are equal partners, 2) families choose their levels of involvement in decision making and implementation, and 3) families are supported in ways that they consider useful. If a consensus is reached on the IFSP after a partnership is established, then there is a better chance that desired outcomes will be achieved (Dunst, Trivette, & Deal, 1988).

Legal Rationale

Partnerships cannot be legislated. Part H of the Individuals with Disabilities Education Act (IDEA) of 1990, PL 101-476, does specify a series of rights and safeguards to ensure parent participation in early intervention. As an introduction to early intervention, parents are often given a set of written procedural safeguards. It is critical that parents be provided these rights and that they understand them. The context and manner in which this information is shared should set the stage for future positive interactions.

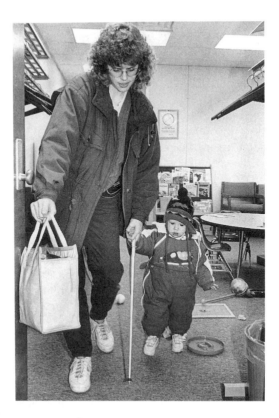

Procedural safeguards are not meant to be used only to resolve adversarial situations. They are a basis for mutual knowledge about the IFSP process and parents' involvement in that process. Legislation makes it clear that parents and service providers are intended to work together throughout the IFSP process. It specifies the following: when parents must receive written notice; when parents must give consent; how parents should be involved in evaluation, programming, and placement; parents' rights to review records; and parents' rights to due process.

Theoretical and Empirical Rationale

The family is the natural context in which infants and toddlers live and grow. Intervention with children affects and includes a family even if that family is not the target of the intervention. "The success of all interventions will rest on the quality of the provider–family relationships, even when the relationship itself is not the focus of the intervention" (Kalmanson & Seligman, 1992, p. 48).

The idea of developing partnerships with families in the early intervention process is grounded in family systems theory and in various ecological models (Guralnick, 1991). Bronfenbrenner's (1979) seminal framework, which comprises the microsystem, mesosystem, exosystem, and macrosystem, has been used as the basis for conceptualizing work with young children from an ecological perspective. His model is useful in identifying sources of environmental influences on development and in understanding the relationships among these influences as they operate at the different levels (i.e., systems) just listed. For instance, the level of the microsystem—the system most frequently targeted in early intervention research—was defined as "a pattern of activities, roles, and interpersonal relations experienced by the developing person in a given setting with particular physical and material characteristics" (Bronfenbrenner, 1979, p. 22). Many recommended practices in early intervention result from the influence of Bronfenbrenner's model.

An appreciation of the transactional nature of interactions and the importance of environments led to the emphasis in Part H on children's natural settings as contexts for evaluation, assessment, and intervention services. In addition, if parents' interactions with their children influence the children's development, then early intervention services should consider the various types of parent–child interactions and the typical daily routines of parents and children. Service providers need to look to parents for information and to observe children in natural settings during daily routines (Guralnick, 1991).

Studies demonstrate that parents' participation in the education of older children results in greater success for the children (Christenson, Rounds, & Franklin, 1992; Epstein, 1987; Powell, 1989; Swap, 1992). Smith and Strain (1988) studied the critical features of effective early intervention and found that parents' involvement resulted in benefits for families and success for their children. Raver (1991) summarized research with families by stating that "Basically, intervention services that focus on increasing parent and family competence appear to produce positive effects on children and families" (p. 11).

Birth-to-3 and Beyond: The Broader Influence of Partnerships

The philosphical foundations of family-centered care highlight the importance of parent and provider partnerships. The skills and knowledge that parents gain in early intervention may assist them in their possibly lifelong efforts to advocate for their children across multiple, complex, and often dysfunctional systems. McGill-Smith (1992) said that parents of young children with special needs need to become the link, or "glue," that holds all of the services together. One hopes these notions inherent in family-centered care will continue to spread across all social, health, education, and political systems.

It is important to think beyond the triad that comprises parents, children, and service providers and to advocate actively for parent–professional partnerships in program planning, development, implementation, and evaluation. Building partnerships with parents and involving them purposefully and meaningfully at multiple levels within the early intervention process while providing them with options regarding their types and degrees of involvement can lead to benefits for children, families, service providers, programs, program administrators, and the community. Including parents' perspectives in all aspects of the process will facilitate the development of family-centered, culturally competent services.

HOW CAN PARTNERSHIPS BE DEVELOPED AND ENHANCED?

Self-Examination of Attitudes About Partnerships

At the core of the process of developing partnerships is attitude (Christenson, 1993). Self-awareness is the most fundamental component of the communication process model (see Chapter 6). A related skill is being aware of one's own communication patterns, past experiences, values, beliefs, needs, goals, abilities to empathize, and listening and responding skills. Similarly, when developing partnerships, one must begin by examining one's attitudes about partnerships. Indeed, the first step is self-assessment: "Participants in partnership must engage in a reflective self-assessment process that examines one's own values and beliefs, expectations, desire for change, and patterns of interactive behaviors" (Paget & Chapman, 1992, p. 266).

Christenson (1993) discussed the following five attitudinal variables that facilitate or mediate home–school partnerships: 1) believing that there is a shared responsibility for the child at school, 2) recognizing everyone's perspectives, 3) using a common language and sharing information, 4) working together to enhance the child's development, and 5) having multiple and flexible options for parents to be involved in ways that are meaningful to them.

These attitudinal variables are useful in early intervention as well. For example, if both the parents and the service providers believe that they have a shared responsibility for a child's outcomes as outlined in the IFSP, then both will contribute information and skills in working to achieve those outcomes. For example, the opportunity to develop a partnership arose when Germaine and Trisha understood their respective perspectives on life, especially those concerning how difficult it is for single parents to raise children with limited financial resources.

ACTIVITY: *Old Scripts*

◆ ◆ ◆

Often our attitudes about the people with whom we work are based on early life experiences. Think back to your family of origin. Write down two or three sayings that you remember your parents using in relationship to others (e.g., "Hard work never hurt anyone," "If you can't say anything nice don't say anything at all"). Examine the sayings that you selected. How might their meanings have influenced how you relate to others? How have they influenced the attitudes you have toward partnerships? ◆

Identifying and Eliminating Barriers to Partnerships

After a thorough self-examination of personal attitudes about working in partnership, it is essential to examine the interdisciplinary team and eliminate chronic attitudes and practices that may hamper the development of partnerships. Some common barriers cited by Salisbury (1992) include the following:

- *Attitudes, perceptions, and values:* insensitivity to differences among families; viewing parents or service providers as adversaries rather than as partners; viewing parents as less perceptive or knowledgeable than service providers; mismatch between parents' and service providers' priorities and expectations
- *Communication:* brochures and evaluation reports not in parents' primary language; service providers' use of jargon without explaining terminology; parents' limitations in reading correspondence (e.g., unclear newsletters from the service program about opportunities for involvement); service providers' limiting communication to administrative tasks or to discussion of problems only; stressful or unpleasant communication between parents and service providers
- *Provider constraints:* lack of knowledge about resources or current literature and trends in early intervention; limited time allotted for meaningful conversations with parents; inadequate organizational abilities of service providers, leading to interference with task follow-up
- *Logistical:* transportation or child care for parents to attend events may not be supported or available; scheduling difficulties; team dynamics may interfere with inclusion of parents

The interdisciplinary team can identify these barriers by using program evaluations and surveys of parents' satisfaction and by noting persistent parent and service provider concerns that arise in the IFSP process. Once a barrier is identified, creative group problem-solving activities can be used, and a plan can be developed, implemented, and evaluated.

Johns and Harvey (1993) suggested that service providers' resistance to working with families in partnership stemmed from three types of sources: organizational, professional, and personal. When service providers are asked to change their attitudes or practices, their reactions may vary. Whatever the case, service providers need to be supported in the process of change. Johns and Harvey (1993) recommended that long-term training programs be offered that incorporate 1) principles of adult learning, 2) a focus on building trust, and 3) an examination of service providers' values and beliefs about families. Because Part H is a relatively new program that is undergoing rapid development and change, programs need to have a means of systematically maintaining and improving program quality over time. In-service training is an effective means of supporting both organizational and individual growth (Trohanis, 1994).

Building Partnership Throughout the IFSP Process

Chapter 4 of this book is devoted to describing the IFSP process and highlighting methods for building partnerships, from making initial contacts to completing the transition from early intervention services. Because numerous, concrete suggestions for building partnerships are provided there, only a few are summarized here:

- Ask parents about the level of involvement they desire at all stages of the IFSP process.
- Verify the parents' desired levels of involvement throughout the process, because families' levels of availability may fluctuate with their personal resources.
- Ask family members about their preferred methods of involvement and communication. These may differ from member to member, even within a single family.
- Ask about best times and locations for interactions and services (i.e., utilize checklists, open-ended questionnaires, conversation, or a combination of methods).
- Get an idea of the families' daily activities, resources, supports, concerns, and priorities, and be mindful that there may be changes that affect children, families, and IFSPs.
- Offer a continuum of choices for involvement. This is not an all-or-none commitment. It is important that choices for involvement be meaningful to individual parents.
- Use a problem-solving format so that parents are always involved in defining issues, developing alternative solutions, devising action plans, and evaluating outcomes.
- Commit program resources to support families to participate in advisory and other program activities.
- Involve willing parents in the process of developing creative ways to encourage parents' participation and involvement in the program.

Vosler-Hunter (1989), through the Family as Allies Project, identified a number of strategies that are useful for parents and service providers:

- *Strategies for parents:* 1) expand your sources of support, 2) keep an open mind, 3) satisfy your need for information, 4) know and act on your rights and responsibilities, 5) take an active role in the services for your child, 6) provide information and offer suggestions, 7) know your limits, and 8) recognize efforts by providers.

- *Strategies for providers:* 1) recognize the uniqueness of every family, 2) keep a focus on family strengths, 3) value and act on the expertise of parents, 4) help parents find support from other parents, 5) be honest about your abilities and limitations, 6) be aware of the demands you place on the families, 7) join with parents to be advocates for their child, and 8) listen.
- *Joint strategies for parents and providers:* 1) critically examine your attitudes and beliefs, 2) obtain information and training that will increase your skills, and 3) remember why you work in partnership.

Initiating Systems Change to Incorporate Partnerships

The Institute for Family-Centered Care (1994) has provided the following guidelines for ensuring that parents' voices are strong and well represented at the policy and program levels:

- Maintain a broad view of collaboration by gathering parents' input from a diverse group of parents using a variety of methods.
- Expand the definition of successful parent involvement so that it takes different levels and types of involvement into account.
- Use innovative ways to identify and recruit families to participate (e.g., talk with present and past participants in the program, solicit ideas from other parents, advertise in locations where people with diverse backgrounds may see or hear the advertisements).
- Look for opportunities to promote parents' involvement in new initiatives and suggest that they get involved on teams in which parents are underrepresented.
- Provide training and support to both parents and service providers because working in partnership is a new skill for both.
- Address logistical barriers comprehensively and creatively.
- Believe that parents' participation is essential and that it will be possible to find solutions to challenges that may arise.

Parental burnout can occur when parents are asked to juggle their already busy schedules because of additional commitments to leadership and systems change. Awareness by service providers that this can occur may help to alleviate some of the stress that parents can feel. Gilkerson (1994) emphasized that parents are acting in dual roles when they participate in leadership activities. They are involved in a public situation, such as a board or committee meeting, but are asked to draw upon their private family experiences. Gilkerson (1994) suggested that the program offer additional incentives to parents who take a lead in systems change: 1) provide compensation, 2) establish parental leave for emergencies or to prevent burnout, 3) explore sharing leadership roles to ease responsibility, 4) offer space and clerical support to parents, 5) encourage parents to set boundaries on what they do, 6) provide parents with the consultation they may need to obtain any additional skills or knowledge to fulfill their leadership roles, and 7) allow time to process the emotional issues that arise.

The Early Intervention Program at the Waisman Center on Mental Retardation and Human Development, University of Wisconsin–Madison, provides a number of examples of how parent–professional partnerships can guide a program and influence the early intervention system within a state. This program includes direct service, in-service, and preservice programs, each of which has realized its commitment to parent–professional partnerships in various ways. These include the following: 1) parents are hired as staff for each project and are integral to the planning, development, implementation, and evaluation of the program; 2) parents are co-instructors for both in-service and preservice courses; 3) parents are offered incentives (e.g., honoraria, travel, child care, lodging, meals) to participate in all project activities; 4) parents are offered a series of opportunities to gain skills and knowledge related to systems change, communication, conflict management, advocacy, the legal and legislative processes, coservice coordination, and presentation enhancement (by telling their families' stories); 5) a directory listing parents who are willing to present the parent perspective in classes is shared with an interdisciplinary faculty from across the state; and 6) parents are members on all advisory committees, and there is a parent advisory review panel that reviews training products.

SUMMARY

This chapter explores parent–professional partnerships, by 1) discussing the elements and myths commonly uncovered when defining partnerships, 2) providing a rationale for fostering partnerships, and 3) listing recommendations for enhancing partnerships in the IFSP process as well as at the programmatic and systems levels. It is argued that although there is no agreed-upon operational definition of partnerships, there is agreement regarding the activities and attitudes that are important in successful partnerships. Partnerships in early intervention seem to have benefits for children and even broader benefits for programs and systems. Therefore, a variety of suggestions for building parent–professional partnerships are offered as well.

DISCUSSION QUESTIONS

◆ ◆ ◆   1. Partnerships need to be mutual. What can be done if you, as a parent or service provider, have tried your best to develop a partnership, but that partnership simply will not materialize?

2. Do you think that it is possible for a parent and a service provider to become too close? If so, how might that closeness affect their relationship?

3. How might working in partnership facilitate better outcomes for children receiving early intervention services?

4. Why is it important for parent–professional partnerships to occur at all levels (i.e., child, IFSP, program, state, national) of the early intervention system? ◆

REFERENCES

American Heritage Desk Dictionary. (1981). Boston: Houghton Mifflin Company.

Bronfenbrenner, U. (1979). *The ecology of human development: Experiments by nature and design.* Cambridge: Harvard University Press.

Christenson, S.L. (1993). *Home and school: Problems for or partners in intervention.* Keynote speech given at the Upper Midwest Summer Institute in School Psychology, Madison, WI.

Christenson, S.L., Rounds, T., & Franklin, M.J. (1992). Home–school collaboration: Effects, issues, and opportunities. In S.L. Christenson & J.C. Conoley (Eds.), *Home–school collaboration: Enhancing children's academic and social competence* (pp. 19–51). Silver Spring, MD: National Association of School Psychologists.

Dunst, C.J., & Paget, K.D. (1991). Parent–professional partnerships and family empowerment. In M. Fine (Ed.), *Collaborative involvement with parents of exceptional children* (pp. 25–44). Brandon, VT: Clinical Psychology Publishing Co.

Dunst, C.J., Trivette, C.M., & Deal, A. (1988). *Enabling and empowering families: Principles and guidelines for practice.* Cambridge, MA: Brookline Books.

Dunst, C.J., Trivette, C.M., & Johanson, C. (1994). Parent–professional collaboration and partnerships. In C.J. Dunst, C.M. Trivette, & A.G. Deal (Eds.), *Supporting and strengthening families: Vol. 1. Methods, strategies, and practices* (pp. 197–211). Cambridge, MA: Brookline Books.

Epstein, J.L. (1987). Toward a theory of family–school connections: Teacher practices and parent involvement. In K. Hurrelmann, F. Kaufmann, & F. Losel (Eds.), *Social interventions: Potential and constraint* (pp. 121–136). New York: deGrayter.

Gilkerson, L. (1994). Supporting parents in leadership roles. *Zero to Three, 14*(4), 23–24.

Goodman, J.F. (1994). "Empowerment" versus "best interests": Client–professional relationships. *Infants and Young Children, 6*(4), vi–x.

Guralnick, M.J. (1991). The next decade of research on the effectiveness of early intervention. *Exceptional Children, 58*(1), 174–183.

Individuals with Disabilities Education Act (IDEA) of 1990, PL 101-476. (October 30, 1990). Title 20, U.S.C. 1400 et seq: *U.S. Statutes at Large, 104,* 1103–1151.

Institute for Family-Centered Care. (1994). Involving families in advisory roles: Eight steps to success. *Advances in Family-Centered Care, 1*(2), 2–6.

Johns, N., & Harvey, C. (1993). Training for work with parents: Strategies for engaging practitioners who are uninterested or resistant. *Infant and Young Children, 5*(4), 52–57.

Kagan, S.L. (1991, January). *Interdisciplinary collaboration.* Paper presented to the Center for Family in Society, University of South Carolina, Columbia.

Kalmanson, B., & Seligman, S. (1992). Family–provider relationships: The basis of all interventions. *Infants and Young Children, 4*(4), 46–52.

McGill-Smith, P. (1992). Parents: The critical team member. *OSERS News in Print, 1*(1), 7–11.

Paget, K.D., & Chapman, S.D. (1992). Home–school partnerships and preschool services: From self-assessment to innovation. In S.L. Christensen & J.C. Conoley (Eds.), *Home–school collaboration: Enhancing children's academic and social competence* (pp. 265–288). Silver Spring, MD: National Association of School Psychologists.

Pletcher, L.C., & Deal, A.G. (1993). Parent–professional partnerships: Common misconceptions. *Messenger, 5*(1), 1–3.

Powell, D.R. (1989). *Families and early childhood programs.* Washington, DC: National Association for the Education of Young Children.

Raver, S.A. (1991). Trends affecting infant and toddler services. In S.A. Raver (Ed.), *Strategies for teaching at-risk and handicapped infants and toddlers: A transdisciplinary approach* (pp. 2–25). New York: MacMillian.

Salisbury, C. (1992). Parents as team members: Inclusive teams, collaborative outcomes. In B. Rainforth, J. York, & C. Macdonald (Eds.), *Collaborative teams for students with severe disabilities: Integrating therapy and educational services* (pp. 43–66). Baltimore: Paul H. Brookes Publishing Co.

Smith, B.J., & Strain, P.S. (1988). Does early intervention help? *ERIC Digest 455,* 1–2.

Swap, S.M. (1992). Parent involvement and success for all children: What we know now. In S.L. Christenson & J.C. Conoley (Eds.), *Home–school collaboration: Enhancing children's academic and social competence* (pp. 53–80). Silver Spring, MD: National Association of School Psychologists.

Trohanis, P.L. (1994). Planning for successful inservice education for local early childhood programs. *Topics in Early Childhood Special Education, 14*(3), 311–332.

Vosler-Hunter, R. (1989). *Changing roles, changing relationships: Parent–professional collaboration on behalf of children with emotional disabilities.* Portland, OR: Families as Allies Project.

4

THE INDIVIDUALIZED FAMILY SERVICE PLAN

The Process

Peggy Rosin

◆◆◆

OBJECTIVES

◆◆◆   By completing this chapter, the reader will

- Learn the legal requirements for participation in and implementation of the individualized family service plan (IFSP) and the IFSP process according to Part H of the Individuals with Disabilities Education Act (IDEA) of 1990, PL 101-476
- Understand the principles upon which the IFSP process is based
- Be able to apply the IFSP process, from establishing initial contacts with eligible children and their families to supporting them to make the transition from early intervention
- Be able to identify families' concerns, priorities, resources, and preferences in developing and implementing IFSPs in family–professional interaction throughout the IFSP process   ◆

The IFSP is the cornerstone of family-centered early intervention services for infants and toddlers with special needs and their families (McGonigel, Johnson, & Kaufmann, 1991). The IFSP, which is required by Part H of IDEA, describes not only a document but a planning process as well. The law specifies the content of the IFSP and imposes some requirements for participation and implementation. The planning process, which should involve the family and service providers, results in the identification of the family's desired outcomes for their child, resources, priorities, and preferences. It is this process surrounding the development of the IFSP that is the focus of this chapter.

The IFSP document is only one component of a process that recognizes the family as the focal point of the early intervention system. In the Galinski family story that follows, it is clear that the way in which service providers react in their first meeting with parents sets the stage for the entire IFSP process. One needs to think beyond the paperwork and assume an expanded view of the IFSP process, one that sees the process as 1) a promise to families, 2) a way to build trusting relationships, 3) a vehicle for empowerment, 4) a mechanism for interagency collaboration, 5) a record of the ongoing relationship between the family and the early intervention system, and 6) a guide to program implementation and evaluation. Each of these components is discussed in turn next.

First, the IFSP process can be viewed as a *promise to families.* The IFSP process should foster a partnership between the family and service providers throughout the family's participation in the early intervention system. McGonigel and Johnson (1991) have stated the following:

> The IFSP is a promise to children and families—a promise that their strengths will be built on, that their needs will be met in a way that is respectful of their beliefs and values, and that their hopes and aspirations will be encouraged and enabled. (p. 1)

Past models of work with children with disabilities and their families have focused on deficits (i.e., service providers point out problems and offer solutions on how to fix them). The family-centered philosophy inherent in the IFSP process asks service providers to see the child first, not the disability, and to recognize and appreciate the child within the family context. All families have strengths and challenges regardless of their children's abilities.

Second, the IFSP process can be a *way to build trusting relationships* with parents as the ultimate decision makers in a consensus-building process among all team members. The initial steps in building a trusting relationship take place during the first contact with the family. DeGangi, Royeen, and Wietlisbach (1993) interviewed both parents and service providers to sort out what they considered to be the critical elements in the IFSP process. Results from both groups indicated that personal characteristics, especially communication skills, were key to effective collaborative relationships. Summers et al. (1990) examined family preferences regarding how service providers gather information. Families preferred that service providers use a conversational style, ask nonintrusive questions, have keen listening skills, and be willing to spend time developing rapport.

There is a mandatory 45-day time limit for completing the IFSP. Some parents and providers may see this as working against building rapport or a healthy relationship. This time frame is intended to ensure that families have expedient access to the services that their children need. Service providers can apply strategies within the process that may help to build trust. Some examples include the following: viewing the

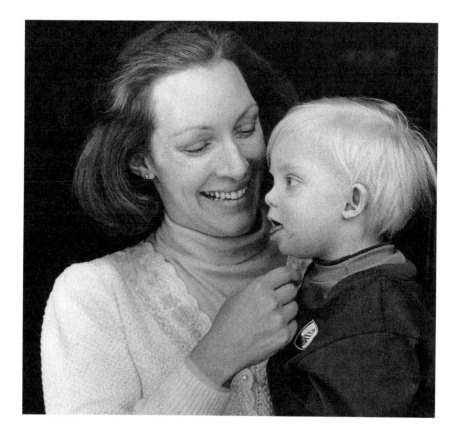

assessment as beginning with the first contact with the family, spending several sessions preparing the parents for the IFSP meeting, and encouraging the parents to invite someone whom they trust to the meetings.

Third, the IFSP process can be a *vehicle for empowerment*. Dunst, Trivette, and Deal (1994) associated the following three assumptions with the concept of empowerment: 1) parents are competent or are capable of becoming competent, 2) opportunities should be created for parents to exhibit competence, and 3) needs should be met in a way that promotes parents' sense of control over their own lives and the lives of their children. The process of developing the IFSP should present opportunities for team problem solving. The primary roles of a service provider are to provide parents with information and to encourage them to be active team members in making decisions about their children's IFSPs. It should be remembered, however, that parents may desire different levels of involvement at different times, depending on their emotional, physical, and financial resources.

The IFSP process is empowering if it builds on a family's strengths and offers needed support at a level that is acceptable to the family. For some families, the service provider may assist in organizing IFSP outcomes into realistic, achievable goals. For example, a parent may set as an outcome learning to read so that he or she can make appointments for his or her child. The long-term goal may be to devise strategies that will assist the parent in learning to read (e.g., providing information about adult literacy programs or tutors). Short-range goals for immediate success might include finding alternative ways of notifying the parent about appointments, arranging assistance in using the library, or locating books on tape. Other families may need little assistance to achieve their desired outcomes. The level of support should be individualized and based on the family's requests.

Fourth, the IFSP process can be used as a *mechanism for interagency collaboration.* During the IFSP process, the family and service provider may need to draw upon both formal and informal resources and services from various agencies to address child and family outcomes. Frequently, one agency is unable to meet the needs of an infant or toddler with special needs and the needs of his or her family. This is especially true if the child has complex medical conditions or multiple developmental delays. Thus, the IFSP specifies who will take responsibility for which portions of the plan.

Fifth, the IFSP process can be viewed as a *record of the ongoing relationship between the family and the early intervention system.* The IFSP document is a record both of conversations among team members and of the decisions made by them. It should be fluid and responsive to ongoing changes in the lives of the child and family.

Sixth, the IFSP process is a *guide to program implementation and evaluation.* The value of the IFSP diminishes if it is not used as a guide to implementation. The IFSP specifies the outcomes that are desired for the child and family, the type and frequency of services, and the resources needed to achieve outcomes. Use of specific curricula may not be successful or appropriate in light of the parents' articulated needs. Periodic review of the IFSP allows for regular opportunities to measure progress toward outcomes. Specific, clear outcomes should be developed and referred to repeatedly. With family outcomes, it is helpful to use phrases such as "in order to" or "so that" to clarify the outcome's relevance to early intervention (e.g., "Mother would like to learn to read in order to keep track of appointments and classes for herself and her child").

Review of IFSP outcomes allows for the evaluation of the plan's success as well. In addition to measuring parents' satisfaction with the early intervention system, evaluation can be useful in tracking outcomes. Agencies can use these data to determine if changes are needed in services provided to children and families.

THE GALINSKI STORY: A CHANGE IN PLANS

Susan and John Galinski waited to have their first baby. They waited until they finished school, got jobs they wanted, bought a house, and saved a little money in the bank. They planned everything very carefully. But they had not planned for their child to be born with Down syndrome. Timmy was born with a heart problem as well, and he needed to have surgery soon after birth. Susan and John were in a state of confused exhaustion during the first 8 months of Timmy's life.

Timmy came through the surgery well. He grew and developed, and he even began to sleep through the night. Susan felt that she was ready to start looking at some of the information on Down syndrome that had piled up, unread, on the desk. She was not sure, however, if she was ready for contact with a birth-to-3 program. The doctors and nurses who had played a major role in her family's lives since Timmy's birth had recommended the birth-to-3 program a few times. Tomorrow she would be taking Timmy to the clinic for a checkup; she knew the suggestion would be made again. She was not sure what she wanted to do, but she wanted to do the right thing. Susan did not want the people at the clinic to think that she did not love Timmy. She did love him, but there had been so many people making suggestions in Timmy's short life.

John was not sure about getting involved in a program either. He was tired of people asking questions and giving advice. He just wanted things to get back to normal. Susan convinced John to at least listen to what the program had to offer. She wanted to ensure that everything would be done to help Timmy reach his potential. She said that she would feel guilty if they missed something important for Timmy's development. John agreed reluctantly to let Susan contact the birth-to-3 program.

Susan called the program the next morning and talked with Jane Morgan. Jane was a service coordinator and teacher with the Gateway birth-to-3 program. Susan and Jane chatted about events that had occurred since Timmy's birth, and Jane set up an appointment to visit the Galinskis' home. Because of Susan's concerns about Timmy's development, Jane suggested that the physical therapist and the speech-language pathologist accompany her to the meeting. Susan hesitated at the prospect of meeting three new people all at once, but agreed. As Susan talked about her life since Timmy's birth, she understood why she was exhausted. She knew that she and John needed a break.

Jane and the other Gateway staff arrived at the Galinski home late as a result of an earlier home visit and appeared rushed. John was at work. Susan welcomed the staff into her home, but when Timmy saw them he started to cry and fuss. As Jane introduced the two staff members, his crying became louder. Jane assured Susan that they were used to crying babies, but Susan was feeling agitated. Jane handed Susan some brochures and began to describe their program and what they had to offer. She added that Susan had certain rights in the process. Susan was having trouble remembering the other two staff members' names. One said that she wanted to play with Timmy on the floor; the other wanted to ask Susan some questions. Timmy was still crying and Susan could not concentrate. She was not sure what to do or say. She wished John were with her.

Jane started talking about how the program was family centered and designed to meet her needs as well as those of John and Timmy. She said that Susan would be a decision maker in the process and asked her what her needs were, but Susan could not begin to try to answer. Right now she wanted Timmy to stop crying and for these women to leave her alone. Maybe she was not ready. Maybe she could not handle anything else—not another thing, not another question. Susan began to cry.

PART H OF IDEA AND THE IFSP PROCESS

While reading this section about the legal requirements of the IFSP process, keep a broad perspective of the process in mind. The law is intended to serve children with special needs and their families, and knowledge of the law is essential. The ultimate goal is to develop early intervention practices that are based on the philosophical underpinnings of the law.

Part H of the Education of the Handicapped Act Amendments of 1986, PL 99-457, added to the Education of the Handicapped Act (EHA) of 1970, PL 91-230, a program designed to encourage states to establish comprehensive, coordinated, family-centered, multidisciplinary, inter-agency systems of early intervention. Part H created a discretionary program to assist states in the planning, development, and implementation of a service system for eligible infants and toddlers from birth to age 3. Subsequently, in October 1990, the EHA was updated and renamed the Individuals with Disabilities Education Act (IDEA) of 1990, PL 101-476. In October 1991, Congress enacted the Individuals with Disabilities Education Act Amendments, PL 102-119, which reauthorized Part H for 3 more years.

Each participating state must phase in a system of early intervention that is suited to the specific needs of the state and encompasses the 14 components mandated by federal law. Table 4.1 lists the necessary components of a statewide comprehensive system of early intervention. The IFSP and service coordination aspects of managing the IFSP process are a legislated component of early intervention for all participating states. Trohanis (1994) reported that as of October 1, 1993, 41 states and jurisdictions were ensuring full implementation, 10 states (plus the District of Columbia and Puerto Rico) were approved for a second year of extended participation, and 1 state (Mississippi) did not apply for funds. The collab-

Table 4.1.   Components of a statewide comprehensive system of early intervention services for infants and toddlers with special needs, including American Indian infants and toddlers

1. Definition of developmentally delayed
2. Time table for ensuring appropriate services to all in need
3. Timely and comprehensive multidisciplinary evaluation of needs of children and families
4. Individualized family service plan and service coordination (case management) services
5. Comprehensive Child-Find and referral system
6. Public awareness program
7. Central directory of services, resources, and research and demonstration projects
8. Comprehensive system of personnel development
9. Single line of authority in a lead agency designated by the governor for carrying out
    a. General administration and supervision
    b. Identification and coordination of all available resources
    c. Assignment of financial responsibility to the appropriate agency
    d. Procedures to ensure services are provided and to resolve intra- and interagency agreements
    e. Entry into formal interagency agreements
10. Policy pertaining to contracting or making arrangements with local service providers
11. Procedure for timely reimbursement of funds
12. Procedural safeguards
13. Policies and procedures for personnel standards
14. System for compiling data on the early intervention programs

From the National Early Childhood Technical Assistance System (NEC★TAS). (1993). *A national reform agenda for services to young children with special needs and their families.* Chapel Hill, NC: Author; reprinted by permision.

orative advocacy efforts of parents, professional organizations, and others played a key role in passing this legislation.

Eligibility

When a child is referred for early intervention, a logical first question is: Is the child eligible for services? An early intervention team, organized by a service coordinator, is responsible for convening a multidisciplinary evaluation to answer this question. The team comprises the child's parent(s) and at least two qualified personnel in the area(s) of concern, frequently representing more than one agency. The team examines all relevant data, including medical records, records of developmental functioning, and records of previous intervention. The team looks at the following five areas of development: 1) cognition; 2) physical development, including motor skills, vision, and hearing; 3) communication; 4) social and emotional development; and 5) adaptive or self-help skills development.

There are three ways in which a child may become eligible for early intervention services. The child may 1) exhibit a developmental delay, as defined by the state; 2) have a diagnosed condition that is likely to result in a developmental delay; or 3) be at risk for developmental delay. Informed clinical opinions at the individual as well as team levels are integral to eligibility determination. Part H mandates that informed clinical opinions be used to safeguard against the use of test scores as the sole measure of eligibility (Biro, Daulton, & Szanton, 1991).

Numerous single-domain and multidomain standardized and criterion-referenced instruments can be used to develop an individualized evaluation protocol to address the developmental concerns about a child. Because a critique of current instruments is beyond the scope of this chapter, the reader is referred to reviews by Hanson and Lynch (1989), McLean and McCormick (1993), Nugent and Davidson (1992), and Taylor (1993).

In the Galinski story, Timmy is eligible for services because he was diagnosed as having Down syndrome. Although there is significant variability in the developmental outcomes for people with Down syndrome, it is a condition typically associated with cognitive and communication disabilities. Therefore, Timmy is considered to be eligible for services based on his diagnosis, and an assessment will be performed to determine his profile of abilities.

Each participating state is responsible for defining *developmental delay.* This is an important and difficult task. How a state defines developmental delay will be the primary factor in determining the number of children who receive services, the types of services provided, and ultimately the cost to the state for providing those services. Many different categories and standards are used throughout the United States to determine a child's eligibility for services. Benn (1993) reported the results of a content analysis regarding states' definitions of developmental delay. Of the 42 states with documented criteria, 38% included test data as the only criterion, 11% relied on professional judgment, and 51% used a combination of both measures. Table 4.2 provides sample definitions used by Arkansas, Colorado, Massachusetts, Ohio, and Wisconsin, each of which has implemented Part H fully (i.e., by providing eligible children and their families with evaluation, assessment, service coordination, IFSP documents, early intervention services, and procedural safeguards).

ACTIVITY: *Defining Who Is Eligible for Early Intervention*

◆ ◆ ◆   Table 4.2 details the eligibility criteria for five states. What is the eligibility criteria for children in your state? Reflecting on the definition for your state answer the following questions:

1.   To determine eligibility in your state, do you need to use a standardized or criterion-referenced measure?
2.   What are some arguments for the use of either type of measure?
3.   Are there some children for whom the use of professional judgment might be the most appropriate method of determining eligibility?   ◆

Table 4.2. Definitions of eligibility

State	Definition of developmental delay	Serving children at risk	Comments
Arkansas	2 standard deviations in one area or 35% delay in months from birth to 18 months; 2 standard deviations in one area, 1.5 standard deviations in two areas, or 25% delay in months from ages 18 to 36 months	Yes (medical/biological)	At risk includes children who have medical conditions known to increase statistical risk for long-term medical and developmental problems, including medical conditions resulting from environmental problems such as failure to thrive or child abuse
Colorado	1.5 standard deviations in one or more areas or equivalent in percentile (7%) or standard scores	Yes (parents with developmental delay)	At risk includes only children of parents with developmental disabilities; will study serving other groups at risk
Massachusetts	Guideline: Developmental delay in one or more areas Age 6 months–1.5 months' delay Age 12 months–3 months' delay Age 18 months–4 months' delay Age 24 months–6 months' delay Age 30 months–7 months' delay	Yes	Biological; environmental requires three or more risk factors; lists of child and family characteristics
Ohio	Child has not reached developmental milestones for chronological age (i.e., a "measurable delay")	No	Will study feasibility of serving children at risk
Wisconsin	25% delay or 1.3 standard deviations in one area; clinical opinion (i.e., decision of multidisciplinary team); atypical development	No	Will study serving children at risk; atypical development defined; list of established conditions, including addiction at birth

Assessment

If the team determines that a child is eligible for services, an assessment follows. According to Part H, assessment involves the initial and ongoing procedures used by family members and qualified personnel to deter-

mine an eligible child's unique needs as well as the nature and extent of
the early intervention services required by that child and his or her family to meet those needs. Fewell (1991) summarized the following five
emerging trends in the assessment of infants and toddlers: 1) play-based
assessment, 2) ecological inventories, 3) arena assessment (i.e., team assessment with a child and family facilitator), 4) adaptive assessment, and
5) assessment that includes parent–child and peer–child interactions.
Many of these naturalistic trends capitalize on assessing a child in a familiar context with familiar people doing familiar activities. The purpose
is to get a valid picture of the child and to include valuable input from
parents and caregivers.

In the Galinski story, Jane might have asked Susan some questions
during their first conversation that could have made the visit go more
smoothly. Questions Jane might have asked include the following:
What's the best time of the day for you and Timmy? How does Timmy
react to strangers? What is the best way to approach Timmy? Do you
want a support person with you when the team convenes?

In addition to the assessment of the child, Part H also incorporates a
family-directed assessment into the IFSP process. The family-directed assessment refers to the ongoing process by which a family and service
providers work in partnership to identify and understand the family's
concerns, resources, and priorities. The family's beliefs and values, as
well as relevant cultural factors, are taken into account. The goals are to
provide services and support and to build the family's capacity to meet
the child's developmental needs (Bailey & Henderson, 1993). There are
no negative consequences for a family who opts to forgo this family-
directed assessment; it is strictly voluntary.

Slentz and Bricker (1992) challenged some current practices related
to family-directed assessments in which interventionists conduct comprehensive assessments of families across a range of functional areas
(e.g., family needs, roles, knowledge, skills, environment, stress, coping
strategies, social supports). The authors argue that the intent of the federal regulations has been overinterpreted, and service providers press for
information that is not mandated clearly for inclusion in the IFSP. Information should be tied directly to identifying a family's resources, priorities, and concerns, and it should relate to enhancing the child's development.

As it relates to families, the term *assessment* is misleading. It is not the
family that needs to be assessed, but rather, how the outcomes of the
IFSP fit the family's context and concerns. Paisley, Irwin, and Tuchman
(1994) characterized the process of identifying a family's concerns, priorities, and resources as follows: 1) it provides family members with an opportunity to explore the ways in which they influence their child's development, 2) it ensures that the IFSP will be appropriate for the family,
3) it gives families options regarding the ways in which their concerns

are identified and addressed, 4) it is confidential, 5) it includes only what family members intend to share, 6) it acknowledges the family's concerns, and 7) it provides a record of the family's experiences.

Services

Early intervention services for an eligible child and his or her family are based on parents' desired outcomes for their child and on the child's developmental needs. Services are provided with the parents' written consent. Together, parents and service providers review the desired outcomes and the menu of options available for working toward those outcomes. Early intervention services may include the following:

- Assistive technology
- Audiology services
- Communication support
- Family education and counseling
- Health care services that will enable the child to benefit from other early intervention services
- Medical services (for diagnostic or evaluative purposes only)
- Nursing
- Nutrition services
- Occupational therapy
- Physical therapy
- Psychological services
- Social work
- Special instruction
- Transportation that will enable the child and family to receive early intervention services
- Vision services

Raab, Davis, and Trepanier (1993) promoted a resource-oriented approach that employs a broad-based definition of support for children and families. As defined by Part H, services may constitute one category of resources. Other categories include the following: economic resources, child care resources, recreation supports, and life necessities. This resource-oriented model includes the following five types of assistance that can be offered to a family who is trying to achieve an outcome: 1) informational support, 2) material aid, 3) instrumental assistance (e.g., time, labor), 4) instructional guidance and feedback, and 5) emotional support. This model discourages the early intervention system, individual programs, and service providers from 1) matching children and families to existing services, and 2) devising IFSPs according to an existing menu of services. Instead, a resource-oriented approach considers a full range of formal and informal resources and methods for meeting the needs of individual children and families.

Content of the IFSP Document

The IFSP document is intended to reflect a fluid process that is responsive to the changing needs of a child and family:

> The IFSP—the written product itself—is possibly the least important aspect of the entire IFSP process. Far more important are the interaction, collaboration, and partnerships between families and professionals that are necessary to develop and implement the IFSP. (McGonigel & Johnson, 1991, p. 1)

Certain elements must be included in a child's IFSP document:

- Information about the child's developmental status, including statements about his or her present levels of ability that are based on professionally acceptable objective criteria
- The basis for the determination of the child's eligibility for early intervention services
- Summaries of the evaluation and the initial assessment of the child, as well as reports of any ongoing assessments
- With the parents' permission, a summary of the family's resources, priorities, and concerns related to enhancing the child's development
- Statements of the expected outcomes for the child and family (as identified by the IFSP team) and of the criteria, procedures, and time lines that will be used to determine progress toward those outcomes (or to determine need for modification of outcomes)
- Information about the frequency and intensity of the early intervention services needed to achieve outcomes; the service delivery model; the setting in which services will be provided; payment arrangements; the projected time frame for initiation and duration of services; and, if appropriate, the medical or other services the child needs that will not be provided by the early intervention program and the steps that will be taken to secure those services
- The name of the service coordinator
- Steps taken to support the family through transitions
- Provisions for ongoing review, evaluation, and, when needed, revision of the plan

Each state is developing its own format for including these elements. In some states, an early intervention program can use either the format suggested by the state or its own format (see Appendix A at the end of this chapter for a sample IFSP form developed by the Bridges for Families Early Intervention program). All of the required elements must be included; however, states or programs may add others. The IFSP should be contained in one folder, and the parents should have a complete copy.

Time Frames for IFSP

The law specifies a time line that must be considered during the IFSP process—determining eligibility for early intervention services and the need for developing, reviewing, and revising the IFSP. These four times are discussed below.

With the parents' permission, the primary referral source has *2 working days* to refer a child for an evaluation from the time the source concludes there is cause to believe the child has a developmental delay or a condition that has a high probability of resulting in a developmental delay. From the day the responsible agency receives the referral, it has *45 days* within which to 1) complete the evaluation and initial assessment, and 2) hold an IFSP meeting to develop a service plan. (Exceptional circumstances may delay the evaluation and initial assessment and therefore the development of the IFSP. In such instances, an interim IFSP is developed in collaboration with the parents.)

After the initial IFSP has been developed, it must be reviewed *every 6 months*. It may be reviewed more frequently if reviews are warranted or requested by the parents. The purposes of such reviews are to determine progress toward desired outcomes and to revise outcomes or services as needed.

At least annually, the service coordinator must convene a meeting to evaluate and revise the IFSP as needed. Unlike the 6-month review, this meeting must include a person involved directly in conducting the evaluation and assessment (see Appendix B at the end of this chapter for a time line overview).

PHILOSOPHICAL FRAMEWORK OF THE IFSP PROCESS

> The individual needs and circumstances of each state and program influence the specific IFSP policies and procedures they choose to adopt. If family-centered early intervention is to become a reality, however, there are a few commonly shared principles that form a framework for IFSP policies and procedures that will enable and empower families as they invite early intervention programs into their lives. (McGonigel, 1991, p. 7)

McGonigel (1991) put forth 10 principles underlying the IFSP process. At the core of these principles is the notion that family-centered early intervention seeks to "build on and promote the strengths and competencies present in all families" (p. 8). These principles[1] are the following:

1. Infants and toddlers are uniquely dependent on their families for their survival and nurturance. This dependence necessitates a family-centered approach to early intervention.

---

[1]These principles are reprinted by permission from McGonigel, M.J. (1991). Philosophy and conceptual framework. In M.J. McGonigel, B.H. Johnson, & R.K. Kaufmann (Eds.), *Guidelines and recommended practices for the individualized family service plan* (2nd ed., pp. 7–14). Bethesda, MD: Association for the Care of Children's Health.

2. States and programs should define "family" in a way that reflects the diversity of family patterns and structures.

3. Each family has its own structure, roles, values, beliefs, and coping styles. Respect for and acceptance of this diversity is a cornerstone of family-centered early intervention.

4. Early intervention systems and strategies must honor the racial, ethnic, cultural, and socioeconomic diversity of families.

5. Respect for family autonomy, independence, and decision making means that families must be able to choose the level and nature of their involvement in early intervention.

6. Family–professional collaboration and partnerships are the keys to family-centered early intervention and to successful implementation of the IFSP process.

7. An enabling approach to working with families requires that professionals reexamine their traditional roles and practices and develop new practices when necessary—practices that promote mutual respect and partnerships.

8. Early intervention services should be flexible, accessible, and responsive to family-identified needs.

9. Early intervention services should be provided according to the normalization principle—that is, families should have access to services provided in as normal a fashion and environment as possible and that promote the integration of the child and family within the community.

10. No one agency or discipline can meet the diverse and complex needs of infants and toddlers with special needs and their families. Therefore, a team approach to planning and implementing the IFSP is necessary.

THE IFSP PROCESS: AN OVERVIEW

Each step in the IFSP process presents opportunities for service providers to interact with families in ways that develop and support partnerships. In the Galinski story, there may have been missed opportunities during initial telephone conversations and face-to-face meetings to establish the parents as decision makers in the IFSP process. But it is never too late to begin. How Jane and the rest of the early intervention team responded to Susan was crucial to beginning the relationship.

ACTIVITY: *Getting Started in the IFSP Process*

◆ ◆ ◆   In the story, A Change in Plans, there may have been some information that Jane, the service coordinator, may have asked Susan during their initial phone conversation that may have helped in making the first home visit less stressful. List three things you wish Jane had asked Susan. How can you get at this information without asking a question? ◆

Initial Contacts with the Family

The IFSP process begins when someone refers the child to be evaluated for eligibility for early intervention services. Referrals may come from a variety of sources. Within any community there may be numerous people or agencies that families approach initially with their concerns.

When the responsible agency receives a referral, it assigns a service coordinator to organize an evaluation. As the early intervention process gets under way, parents may choose another service provider (i.e., someone else with whom they have developed a relationship and share more common ground) to act as the service coordinator. The law does not require that parents be allowed to choose their service coordinator; this is a suggested recommended practice. The service coordinator will have a major role throughout the IFSP process.

These first contacts are essential to initiating the partnership between the family and the service system. The process of learning about a family's hopes and preferences for their child in relation to the IFSP process can begin during these initial contacts. Family members can be given information about resources that may help them to develop an agenda. From the outset, the message to the family should be, "We are here for you, and we want to respond to your concerns, priorities, resources, and strengths."

Evaluation and Assessment Planning

Planning the evaluation and assessment of the child provides an important opportunity to establish the parents as decision makers in the IFSP process. A discussion with the family helps to set the agenda for evaluation and assessment. A variety of tools are available to structure meetings with parents and to help parents clarify the outcomes that they want for their child. Recommended resources (listed by subject matter) include the following:

- *Early Intervention—Tailor Made* (Kjerland & Eide, 1990)
- *McGill Action Planning System* (Forest & Lusthaus, 1989)
- *Circle of Friends* (Perske, 1988)
- *Personal Futures Planning* (Mount & Zwernik, 1988)
- *Eco Maps* (McGonigel et al., 1991)

The process of evaluation and assessment is full of opportunities for strengthening the partnership between parents and service providers. The evaluation of the child to determine eligibility for early intervention should consider information from multiple sources, evaluate multiple developmental domains, and use multiple procedures to address concerns. Meisels and Provence (1989) cited the following recommended practices[2] for evaluation and assessment:

- Evaluation and assessment are parts of the intervention process.
- Collaboration with, and informed consent of, families are integral to the process.
- The process must reflect sensitivity to cultural diversity.
- Procedures used must be reliable and valid for children and must consider their sensorimotor capabilities and cultural background.
- Instruments should be used only for their specified purposes.
- Multiple sources of information should be used. Information should span a continuum of contexts that is determined by families' concerns, children's characteristics, and the availability of appropriate procedures and instruments.
- The more familiar and relevant the procedures are to specific children, the more likely it is that the results will be reliable.
- Screening should not be the only activity that initiates the IFSP process; children with diagnosed conditions that are likely to result in developmental delays are eligible for early intervention services.
- The periodic reevaluations called for in the time line of the IFSP process are essential because of the rapid developmental changes that occur in infants and toddlers.
- Professionals involved in the IFSP process need to have specific skills, knowledge, and attitudes related to infant and toddler development, family-centered intervention, and collaborative interdisciplinary and interagency team building.

Mendenhall (1990) suggested structuring family-centered evaluation and assessment around the following questions, which should be answered during the evaluation and assessment process:

- *Team composition:* Who will be included on the evaluation and assessment team?
- *Content:* What will be evaluated and assessed?
- *Plan:* How will evaluation and assessment be conducted?
- *Implementation:* What actually happened during evaluation and assessment?
- *Interpretation:* What does all the information gathered mean?
- *Application:* How are the data going to be used?

Throughout the evaluation and assessment of the child, information is given to family members so that they can make informed decisions in

---

[2]Recommended practices from Meisels, S.J., & Provence, S. (1989). *Screening and assessment: Guidelines for identifying young disabled and developmentally vulnerable children and their families.* (A Report of the National Early Childhood Technical Assistance System). Washington, DC: ZERO TO THREE/National Center for Clinical Infant Programs.

Table 4.3.   Building parent–professional partnerships

Before evaluation and assessment

- Obtain parents' consent in writing prior to initial evaluation and assessment.
- Explain the process and procedural safeguards.
- Ask whether an interpreter is needed if a family's first language is not English.
- Offer suggestions to the family about how they might prepare for assessment.
- Determine a location for evaluation and assessment. If the evaluation and assessment will be center based, discuss things to bring (e.g., toys, clothes, snacks).
- Discuss time options (i.e., options that are best for the child and family).
- Discuss possible roles for the family, and determine how they want to participate.
- Ask parents to think about their goals, desired outcomes, and dreams. (The McGill Action Planning System [Forest & Lusthaus, 1990] is an example of a process that can assist parents in preparing for evaluation and assessment.)
- Ask parents to fill out preassessment surveys in their areas of concern.
- Ask parents if they want others (e.g., advocates, friends, relatives) involved in the evaluation and assessment process or during meetings.
- Ask parents if there are other settings in which their child should be observed.
- Ask parents to describe their child's preferences regarding materials (e.g., toys, snacks).
- Ask parents how they think their child's best behaviors might be elicited (e.g., structuring the environment, presenting toys, assigning motor and visual tasks).
- Elicit parents' concerns and preferences.
- Discuss who will be involved in the evaluation and assessment and why.
- Ask parents if siblings will attend evaluation and assessment meetings and whether they would like child care to be provided.
- If parents ask questions to which the professional does not have answers, explain how the evaluation and assessment might answer the questions or that answers may otherwise be available from other sources. Be prepared, however, to acknowledge that answers sometimes are not known.
- Encourage parents to ask specific questions about their child's development.
- Explain to parents that discussions can occur in a variety of settings and that information can be gathered using a variety of methods.

During evaluation and assessment

- Respect parents' preferences concerning times, locations, and desired levels of participation.
- Discuss the evaluation and assessment protocol and how it addresses parents' concerns.
- Explain tests, instruments, and methods as they are presented.
- Ask parents if the child's behavior is typical.
- Before administering a standardized test, explain the parents' roles to maintain standardization.
- Encourage parents to ask questions.
- Ask parents if the child's behavior indicates that a change in tasks or a break is needed.
- If jargon and acronyms are used, explain their meanings.
- Use person-first language (e.g., refer to a child with Down syndrome, not a Down syndrome child).

After evaluation and assessment

- Invite and encourage parents to speak first, ask questions, and make comments.

(*continued*)

Table 4.3.   (*continued*)

- Ask parents whether they feel that the evaluation and assessment process was valid. If they do not think that it was valid, find out why. Ask what was not observed or elicited.
- Provide immediate feedback regarding the evaluation and assessment process to the maximum extent possible.
- Focus on a family's resources rather than deficits.
- Address parents' concerns clearly, even if all their questions were not answered.
- Ask parents how they would like to receive feedback and organize staffing (e.g., one person talks and others offer support or answer questions). Find out the level of detail (e.g., test scores, standard scores, age equivalencies) that the parents would like.
- Use visual and/or graphic tools, not just words, to present information.
- Do not use jargon without explaining it.
- Write reports using person-first language.
- Use a circle of support rather than traditional staffing (Mount & Zwernik, 1988).
- Ask parents about next steps. Ask if and when they would like to meet with either the team as a whole or specific team members to follow up on issues that have not been resolved.
- Ask parents if they have additional questions. Find out if there were things discussed that were not clear or that do not accurately reflect their child as they see him or her.
- Discuss with parents when they will receive written reports.
- Provide the parents with one or two concrete suggestions regarding their concerns.

addressing the preceding questions. Table 4.3 suggests ways to facilitate the development of partnerships between parents and service providers before, during, and after the evaluation and assessment process.

Identification of a Family's Concerns, Priorities, and Resources

As already noted, a family-directed assessment is voluntary. Unless the term *assessment* is carefully explained, it can be misleading to families. Therefore, it is especially important to explain the purpose for asking questions that may seem unrelated to the child.

Beckman and Bristol (1991) warned that the evaluation and assessment process is likely to be perceived as intrusive to the extent that the questions asked are unrelated to 1) the family's concerns, 2) the expressed purpose of the professional's involvement, or 3) the services that will be provided for the family.

The family systems, family development, and family adaptation and adjustment perspectives (see Chapter 2) suggest the types of information that are helpful in getting to know families. Hanft (1991) provided guidelines for service providers to consider when selecting written instruments to use in identifying a family's concerns, priorities, and resources. She stated that each instrument should

- Provide information to assist the family.
- Identify the family's concerns, priorities, and resources rather than state the nature of marital relationships or family dynamics.
- Be appropriate for diverse cultures.
- Be responsive to the family's changing needs.

- Be easily understood in terms of readability and the response format.
- Request information while respecting the family's privacy.
- Be valid and reliable.

Bailey (1991) stated that research and common sense suggest that the procedures for gathering information about a family's concerns, priorities, and resources will vary from family to family. Similarly, an individual family may choose different approaches in the course of several meetings. Being self-aware and listening and responding are important in conversations with families throughout the IFSP process. Several tools for determining parents' concerns, priorities, and resources are listed in Table 4.4.

ACTIVITY: *Methods for Determining Parents' Concerns, Priorities and Resources*

◆ ◆ ◆   Table 4.4 has three categories of options for determining families' concerns, priorities, and resources. Think about your own communication and interaction style and answer the following:

1. Which one of the three general options would you be most comfortable in using and why?
2. How might you adapt a method not as comfortable to you and why might it be important in your work with families?   ◆

Table 4.4.   Tools for determining parents' concerns, priorities, and resources

Verbal interactions
- Interviews—following a predetermined format or style (e.g., the Family Assessment Interview Guide [Turnbull & Turnbull, 1986])
- Conversations—having face-to-face informal contacts or making telephone calls
- Brainstorming—generating many ideas about a topic
- Stories and anecdotes—sharing meaningful occurrences
- Parent-to-parent contact—learning from others' experiences

Written instruments
- Checklists—informal menus of services (e.g., program developing its own checklist or adapting an existing one)
- Scales—priority ratings of needs for a family (e.g., the Family Needs Scale [Dunst, Cooper, Weeldreyer, Snyder, & Chase, 1988])
- Surveys—(e.g., the Family Needs Survey [Bailey & Simeonsson, 1990] and the Parent Needs Survey [Seligman & Benjamin Darling, 1989])
- Questionnaires—lists of questions to be answered by the family (e.g., *How Can We Help?* [Child Development Resources, 1988])

Graphic instruments
- Videotapes, artwork, and photo albums
- Guided team strategies (e.g., the McGill Action Planning System [Forest & Lusthaus, 1989], personal futures planning [Mount & Zwernik, 1988])
- Charting or pictorial tools (e.g., Eco Maps [McGonigel et al., 1991])

Collaborative Development of IFSP Outcomes

Part H of IDEA requires that an IFSP include outcomes expected to be achieved for the infant or toddler and the family. An IFSP outcome is defined as a statement of the changes family members want to see for their child or themselves. The term *outcome* is used instead of *goal* or *objective*—the terms used in individualized education programs and many other service plans. This changed terminology reflects an intended change in practice that is based on family-centered principles. An outcome should be developed as a result of collaboration between parents and service providers.

A collaborative relationship is initiated when the IFSP process begins. By the time the family and service providers are ready to develop outcomes, family members have had ample opportunity to talk about what they want for their child. Service providers are responsible for helping the family to understand information so that they feel confident as collaborators in making decisions.

At least two critical questions must be considered in developing outcomes: 1) What are the different types of outcomes that might be included in an IFSP? and 2) How are the outcomes to be written? Beckman and Bristol (1991) proposed that outcomes be determined by whether the family or the child is the primary recipient of services.

Types of Outcomes

Child-Related Child Outcomes   Child-related child outcomes pertain to specific skills or abilities (e.g., motor, communication, social) of the child. Examples of child outcomes include the following:

- "Marie will learn how to use a hand-to-mouth pattern so that she can feed herself."
- "Tyler will learn to play with at least five different toys so that he can entertain himself independently."

Family-Related Child Outcomes   Family-related child outcomes are related to a family's need for changes in the child (e.g., sleeping or feeding behaviors) that will affect the pleasantness of family life. The following are some examples of family-related child outcomes:

- "We would like to know what Cody means when he cries or makes noises."
- "Our family would like the equipment necessary to take Shawna to visit our friends' and relatives' homes."

Child-Related Family Outcomes   Child-related family outcomes are related to a family's needs. Intervention (e.g., respite care, support groups for family members) focuses on the family rather than on the child. Examples of child-related family outcomes include the following:

* "We would like information about guardianship and wills so that Juanita will be taken care of in case something happens to us."
* "I would like to know about adult reading classes so that I can learn to read information about helping Phillip."

General Family Outcomes General family outcomes are related directly to a family's needs (e.g., eliminating substance abuse, obtaining marital counseling). Examples include the following:

* "I would like information about support groups for single mothers."
* "Because we are new to this community, we would appreciate information about resources for families with young children."

Of course, a change in any family member that results from working toward any of these outcome types will affect the whole family system.

Writing Outcomes

The second question concerns the writing of outcomes. Outcomes written in "behavioral language" (e.g., "The mother will attend a support class once a month for the next 6 months") can add to the pressure on a family. Some families prefer that outcomes regarding family members be written as suggestions: "We talked about three support groups that other families have found helpful. Please call Joan if you'd like more information about any of these groups." (See Appendix C at the end of this chapter for an overview of the five steps to developing an IFSP.)

Implementation of the IFSP

According to Dunst (1991): "Implementation translates the written IFSP into action. Implementation refers to the processes, methods, and procedures used to attain IFSP outcomes" (p. 67). Families are key players in this process. The principles underlying the IFSP process stress that families should be active decision makers in implementing the IFSP. Implementation should promote and strengthen families. Dunst (1991) also listed six conditions essential for implementing the IFSP in a manner consistent with the underlying principles of the IFSP process. Service providers should:

1. Forge family–professional partnerships.
2. Be responsive to changing family concerns.
3. Build on family strengths.
4. Agree upon the strategies to be used in achieving the desired outcomes of the IFSP.
5. Accommodate changes in the implementation of the IFSP with an attitude of flexibility.
6. Encourage family members to determine their desired level of involvement in the implementation of the IFSP. (p. 67)

The service coordinator will have a major role in coordinating the efforts of early intervention team members to achieve IFSP outcomes.

Evaluation of the IFSP and IFSP Process

As discussed previously, there are time frames designated by law for review and evaluation of an IFSP. These time frames should be seen as minimum requirements. It is imperative that the IFSP process be flexible and responsive to the needs of the child and family. A change in the child's or family's status may necessitate a revision of the IFSP before one is required. The IFSP process should be altered to accommodate any resulting change in desired outcomes as well.

Transitions

Some children and families may experience multiple transitions while participating in early intervention. Common transitions that may occur for infants and toddlers with special needs are 1) moving from a neonatal intensive care unit to home, 2) changing from one early intervention program or agency to another, 3) changing service or child care providers, 4) being relocated because of a family move, and 5) leaving the early intervention system. These transitions may be precipitated by such factors as the child's age, health needs, readiness, eligibility, and the family's geographic location or preferences (Rosenkoetter, Hains, & Fowler, 1994).

In the IFSP process, attention is paid to the transitions that a child and family encounter. The service coordinator is responsible for including a transition plan in the IFSP as well as for supporting the child and family during each transition. (See Chapter 10 for detailed descriptions of many of the procedures and strategies employed in the transition process.)

SUMMARY

This chapter emphasizes the IFSP as a process rather than as simply a document describing the service needs of an eligible child and family. The process should be viewed as a series of opportunities for building relationships with a family that recognizes that family's resources and promotes the family as a decision maker for their child. The IFSP process encourages interagency collaboration and provides a means of documenting, implementing, and evaluating the early intervention services provided for a child and his or her family.

Part H of IDEA regulates the aspects of the process that relate to eligibility; evaluation and assessment; services; components of the IFSP document; and time frames for the IFSP document's development, evaluation, and review. It is essential that service providers working in early intervention understand the federal and state mandates that drive the

IFSP process. It is equally important that professionals and programs embrace a family-centered, culturally competent, team-based philosophy as the foundation of all services for children and families. Therefore, an overview of the IFSP process that highlights some strategies for facilitating partnerships with families is also presented.

After completing this chapter, the reader may wish to revisit the Galinski story with more ideas about how to initiate the IFSP process; encourage parents to participate in evaluation and assessment; assist a family in identifying their concerns, priorities, and resources; and develop, implement, and evaluate collaborative IFSP outcomes.

DISCUSSION QUESTIONS

◆ ◆ ◆

1. What advice might you give to Jane before she responds to Susan's crying in the Galinski story?
2. What characteristics of the IFSP process support family-centered practices in early intervention?
3. Why might collaborative development of an IFSP encourage conscientious follow-through by participants?
4. How might you defend the position that the IFSP document is less important than the overall process?
5. Do you think there should be limits in determining a family's needs during the development of an IFSP? If so, how do you determine these limits? If not, how will services to address needs be paid for? Who will assist the family in meeting their needs? ◆

REFERENCES

Bailey, D. (1991). Issues and perspectives on family assessment. *Infants and Young Children, 4*(1), 27–34.

Bailey, D., & Henderson, L. (1993). Traditions in family assessment: Toward an inquiry-oriented, reflective model. In D.M. Bryant & M.A. Graham (Eds.), *Implementing early intervention: From research to effective practice*. New York: Guilford Press.

Bailey, D., & Simeonsson, R. (1990). Family Needs Survey (rev.). In M.J. McGonigel, B.H. Johnson, & R.K. Kaufmann (Eds.), *Guidelines and recommended practices for the individualized family service plan* (2nd ed., pp. D3–D4). Bethesda, MD: Association for the Care of Children's Health.

Beckman, P.J., & Bristol, M.M. (1991). Issues in developing the IFSP: A framework for establishing family outcomes. *Topics in Early Childhood Special Education, 11*(3), 19–31.

Benn, R. (1993). Conceptualizing eligibility for early intervention services. In D.M. Bryant & M.A. Graham (Eds.), *Implementing early intervention: From research to practice* (pp. 18–45). New York: Guilford Press.

Biro, P., Daulton, D., & Szanton, E. (December 30, 1991). Informed clinical opinion. *NEC•TAS Notes* (No. 4). Chapel Hill, NC: National Early Childhood Technical Assistance System.

Child Development Resources. (1988). *How can we help?* Lightfoot, VA: Author.

DeGangi, G., Royeen, C., & Wietlisbach, S. (1993). How to examine the IFSP process: Preliminary findings and a procedural guide. *Infants and Young Children, 5*(2), 42–56.

Dunst, C. (1991). Implementation of the individualized family service plan. In M.J. McGonigel, B.H. Johnson, & R.K. Kaufmann (Eds.), *Guidelines and recommended practices for the individualized family service plan* (2nd ed., pp. 67–78). Bethesda, MD: Association for the Care of Children's Health.

Dunst, C., Cooper, C., Weeldreyer, K., Snyder, K., & Chase, J. (1988). Family Needs Scale. In C. Dunst, C. Trivette, & A. Deal (Eds.), *Enabling and empowering families: Principles and guidelines for practice* (pp. 149–151). Cambridge, MA: Brookline Books.

Dunst, C., Trivette, C., & Deal, A. (1994). Enabling and empowering families. In C. Dunst, C. Trivette, & A. Deal (Eds.), *Supporting and strengthening families: Vol. 1. Methods, strategies and practices* (pp. 2–11). Cambridge, MA: Brookline Books.

Education of the Handicapped Act (EHA) of 1970, PL 91-230. (April 13, 1970). Title 20, U.S.C. 1400 et seq: *U.S. Statutes at Large, 84,* 121–195.

Education of the Handicapped Act Amendments of 1986, PL 99-457. (October 8, 1986). Title 20, U.S.C. 1400 et seq: *U.S. Statutes at Large, 100,* 1145–1177.

Fewell, R. (1991). Trends in the assessment of infants and toddlers with disabilities. *Exceptional Children, 58*(2), 166–173.

Forest, M., & Lusthaus, E. (1989). Promoting educational equality for all students: Circles and maps. In S. Stainback, W. Stainback, & M. Forest (Eds.), *Educating all students in the mainstream of regular education* (pp. 43–57). Baltimore: Paul H. Brookes Publishing Co.

Hanft, B. (1991). *Identification of family resources, concerns, and priorities within the IFSP process.* Baltimore: Governor's Office for Children, Youth, and Families.

Hanson, M., & Lynch, E. (1989). Assessing children and identifying family strengths and needs. In M. Hanson & E. Lynch (Eds.), *Early intervention: Implementing child and family services for infants and toddlers who are at-risk or disabled.* Austin, TX: PRO-ED.

Individuals with Disabilities Education Act (IDEA) of 1990, PL 101-476. (October 30, 1990). Title 20, U.S.C. 1400 et seq: *U.S. Statutes at Large, 104,* 1103–1151.

Individuals with Disabilities Education Act Amendments of 1991, PL 102-119. (October 7, 1991). Title 20, U.S.C. 1400 et seq: *U.S. Statutes at Large, 105,* 587–608.

Kjerland, L., & Eide, K.C. (1990). *Early intervention—tailor made.* Eagan, MN: Project Dakota Outreach.

McLean, M., & McCormick, K. (1993). Assessment and evaluation in early intervention. In W. Brown, S.K. Thurman, & L.F. Pearl (Eds.), *Family-centered early intervention with infants and toddlers: Innovative cross-disciplinary approaches* (pp. 43–79). Baltimore: Paul H. Brookes Publishing Co.

McGonigel, M.J. (1991). Philosophy and conceptual framework. In M.J. McGonigel, B.H. Johnson, & R.K. Kaufmann (Eds.), *Guidelines and recommended practices for the individualized family service plan* (2nd ed., pp. 7–14). Bethesda, MD: Association for the Care of Children's Health.

McGonigel, M.J., & Johnson, B.H. (1991). An overview. In M.J. McGonigel, B.H. Johnson, & R.K. Kaufmann (Eds.), *Guidelines and recommended practices for the individualized family service plan* (2nd ed., pp. 1–5). Bethesda, MD: Association for the Care of Children's Health.

McGonigel, M.J., Johnson, B.H., & Kaufmann, R.K. (Eds.). (1991). *Guidelines and recommended practices for the individualized family service plan* (2nd ed.). Bethesda, MD: Association for the Care of Children's Health.

Meisels, S.J., & Provence, S. (1989). *Screening and assessment: Guidelines for identifying young disabled and developmentally vulnerable children and their families.* Chapel Hill, NC: National Early Childhood Technical Assistance System.

Mendenhall, J. (1990). *Family-centered assessment: Six central elements.* Eagan, MN: Project Dakota Outreach.

Mount, B., & Zwernik, K. (1988). *It's never too early, it's never too late: A booklet about personal futures planning.* St. Paul, MN: Metropolitan Council.

National Early Childhood Technical Assistance System (NEC*TAS). (1993). *A national reform agenda for services to young children with special needs and their families.* Chapel Hill, NC: Author.

Nugent, J.K., & Davidson, C.E. (1992). Newborn and infant assessment. In E. Vazquez-Nuttall, I. Romero, & J. Kalesnik (Eds.), *Assessing and screening preschoolers.* Newton, MA: Allyn & Bacon.

Olson, P.P., & Hains, A.H. (1992). Birth to three time line. In S. Robbins (Ed.), *Toward parent and professional partnership: Guidelines for Wisconsin's individualized family service plan* (p. 7). Madison, WI: Division of Community Services.

Paisley, R., Irwin, L., & Tuchman, L. (1994). *Identifying family concerns, priorities, and resources: Information for early intervention teams.* Madison: University of Wisconsin—Madison, Wisconsin Personnel Development Project.

Perske, R. (1988). *Circle of friends: People with disabilities and their friends enrich the lives of one another.* Nashville: Abingdon Press.

Raab, M., Davis, M., & Trepanier, A.M. (1993). Resources versus services: Changing the focus of intervention for infants and young children. *Infants and Young Children, 5*(3), 1–11.

Rosenkoetter, S.E., Hains, A.H., & Fowler, S.A. (1994). *Bridging early services for children with special needs and their families: A practical guide for transition planning.* Baltimore: Paul H. Brookes Publishing Co.

Seligman, M., & Benjamin Darling, R. (1989). Parent needs survey. In M.J. McGonigel, B.H. Johnson, & R.K. Kaufmann (Eds.), *Guidelines and recommended practices for the individualized family service plan* (2nd ed., pp. D7–D8). Bethesda, MD: Association for the Care of Children's Health.

Slentz, K.L., & Bricker, D. (1992). Family-guided assessment for IFSP development: Jumping off the family assessment bandwagon. *Journal of Early Intervention, 16*(1), 11–19.

Summers, J.A., Dell'Oliver, C., Turnbull, A.P., Benson, H.A., Santelli, E., Campbell, J., & Siegel-Causey, E. (1990). Examining the individualized family service plan process: What are the family and practitioners' preferences? *Topics in Early Childhood Special Education, 10*(1), 78–99.

Taylor, R.L. (1993). Instruments for screening, evaluation, and assessment of infants and toddlers. In D.M. Bryant & M.A. Graham (Eds.), *Implementing early intervention: From research to effective practice.* New York: Guilford Press.

Trohanis, P. (1994). Continuing positive changes through implementation of IDEA. In L.J. Johnson, R.J. Gallagher, M.J. LaMontagne, & J.B. Jordon, J.J. Gallagher, P.L. Hutinger, & M.B. Karnes (Eds.), *Meeting early intervention challenges: Issues from birth to three.* Baltimore: Paul H. Brookes Publishing Co.

Turnbull, A.P., & Turnbull, H.R. (1986). *Families, professionals, and exceptionality: A special partnership.* Columbus, OH: Charles E. Merrill.

Appendix A

IFSP Sample Forms ◆◆◆

The following sample IFSP form is from the Bridges for Families Early Intervention program at the Waisman Center of the University of Wisconsin in Madison, Wisconsin. IFSP forms can vary in format and structure from state to state, and in some states, from program to program. There are mandatory elements (see Content of the IFSP Document in this chapter) that must be included in any set of forms comprising an IFSP. As this chapter stresses, however, it is the process of how the information is collected that is crucial. Also, the language should be family friendly and individualized to reflect the specific child and family for whom it is written.

Individualized Family Service Plan (IFSP)

for: _____ _____ _____ Birthdate: _____ Sex: _____
      (First)   (Middle)   (Last)

Parent(s)/Guardian(s): _____

Address: _____
_____

Telephone: _____ _____'s (work)
            (home)

Social Security #: _____

Physician: _____

Clinic: _____ Insurance: _____
                         Provider

Phone: _____

Early Intervention Service Providers

Name   Role   Agency   Address   Phone   Location   Frequency   Funding

Other People + Agencies Involved with Family
(family members, friends, daycare, community services, specialists, doctors, nurse, others)

Name   Relationship   Address   Phone

_____'s History

... Suggestions :

pregnancy and birth
growth and development
medical information
description of your child
other relevant information

_____'s Development

Date: _____

health: _____

sensory: _____

communication: _____

social-emotional: _____

motor: _____

cognition: _____

self-help: _____

evaluation tool(s): _____

is eligible based on: _____

Family Information

date	Strengths and resources	date	Concerns and priorities

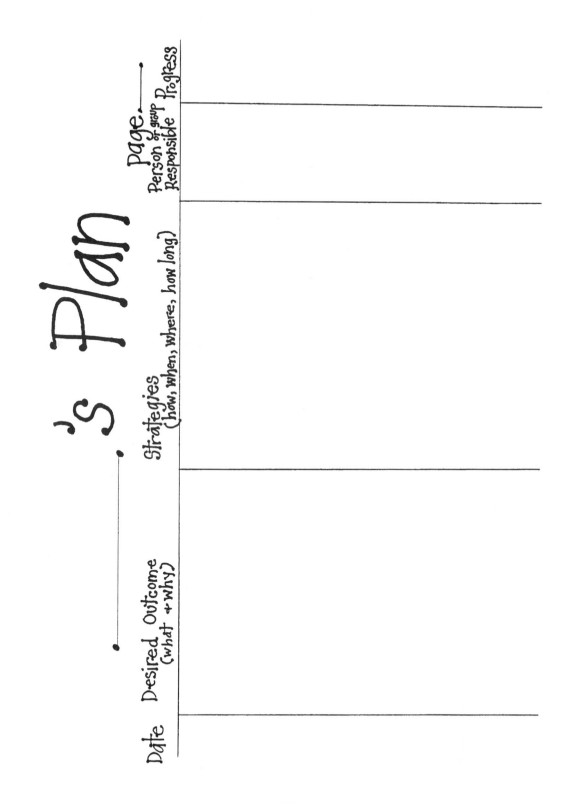

_____'s Plan

Date	Desired Outcome (what + why)	Strategies (how, when, where, how long)	Person or group Responsible	Progress

Page ____

We have worked on this plan and agree that it reflects our goals for _____ and give consent for services described in this plan.

_____'s Team

team member	role	signature	date	date	date
	parent/guardian				
	parent/guardian				
	service coordinator				

Dates

Referral: _____ Evaluation: _____ Services begin: _____

IFSP: _____ update: _____ update: _____ update: _____ transition: _____

Appendix B

Birth-to-3 Time Line ◆◆◆

2 DAYS

Primary referral:

- Request formal screening.
- Conduct formal screening as soon as possible.

If needs are identified, inform parent prior to referral and document method of notification.

Refer for evaluation.

45 DAYS

Agency receipt of referral:

Assign service coordinator.

Begin individualized family service plan (IFSP)→May develop interim IFSP/service coordination.

Have parent-directed discussion of their concerns and priorities; parents consent to evaluate and assess child is obtained.

Evaluation:

- Parent–professional consultation.
- Review existing records.
- Developmental testing.

Determination of eligibility:

- If no, offer to rescreen, provide information on community services, and assist referral.
- If yes, continue with assessment.

Evaluate findings and conclusions.

Child- and family-directed assessment:

- Developmental assessment of child.
- Family strengths, resources, concerns, priorities.

IFSP meeting held to develop service plan.

- Prioritize and plan services.

Provide early intervention services under PL 99-457, Part H.

The time line provided in this appendix is reprinted by permission from Olson, P.P., & Hains, A.H. (1992). Birth to three time line. In S. Robbins (Ed.), *Toward parent and professional partnership: Guidelines for Wisconsin's individualized family service plan* (p. 7). Madison, WI: Division of Community Services.

Appendix C

How Do We Develop an Individualized Family Service Plan? ◆ ◆ ◆

FIRST—Establish a partnership with family.

- For example:
    - Actively listen and share something of yourself.
    - Recognize, respect, and affirm family values, customs, and beliefs.
    - Communicate clearly, openly, and honestly.
    - Continue building the relationship.

SECOND—Gather general information about the child and family.

- For example:
    - Start with the family's perspective about their child with special needs and their family (if they choose).
    - Use creative approaches for gathering information such as conversations, chats, story telling, and brainstorming in addition to traditional strategies, such as interviews.

THIRD—Gather information on the child's present level of development.

- For example:
    - Identify family preferences for involvement in gathering and exchanging information (conduct preassessment planning with family).
    - Conduct formal and informal evaluation assessments as shaped by the family priorities and information needs, as well as child characteristics and diagnostic concerns.
    - Use family language and avoid jargon in order to enable families to participate fully as part of the team.

The material provided in this appendix is reprinted by permission of Olson, P.P., & Hains, A.H. (1992). In S. Robbins (Ed.), *Toward parent and professional partnership: Guidelines for Wisconsin's individualized family service plan* (p. 16). Madison, WI: Division of Community Services.

FOURTH—Identify family strengths, resources, concerns, and priorities based on the family's determination of which aspects of their life are relevant to the child's development. *(NOTE: Inclusion of family information in the IFSP is voluntary on the part of families.)*

- For example:
  - Provide multiple and continuing opportunities to identify their strengths, resources, concerns, and priorities.
  - Provide a broad array of formal and informal options for families to choose from in determining how they will identify their strengths, resources, concerns, and priorities.
  - Respect confidentiality of family-shared information.
  - Honor family-identified information—a concern exists only if the family perceives that the concern exists.

FIFTH—Develop the IFSP including outcomes, strategies, activities, services, and time lines so that the plan reflects the priorities and values of the family.

- For example:
  - Use a collaborative team (family and professionals) process to develop the plan.
  - Respect the family's choices for the level and nature of the involvement of early intervention in their lives.
  - Use resources and services that reflect a range of options and that respond to the family's concerns, priorities, and resources.
  - Use community-based resources and services that are, to the extent possible, provided in locations and times convenient to the family.

SIXTH—Implement and evaluate the IFSP process and plan.

- For example:
  - Provide service coordination to reflect the intent of the IFSP.
  - Provide multiple opportunities and methods for families to evaluate the IFSP process as well as the extent to which outcomes are achieved or concerns are met.
  - Evaluate the comprehensive, coordinated, interdisciplinary, and interagency system from family, staff, and administrative perspectives.

Note: These components of the IFSP process follow a general sequence; however, some steps repeat themselves, some activities are ongoing, and some events are interchangeable.

II

THE EARLY INTERVENTION TEAM
Transdisciplinary and Interagency

◆ ◆ ◆

5

The Team and Models of Teaming

Linda I. Tuchman

◆◆◆

OBJECTIVES

◆ ◆ ◆   By completing this chapter, the reader will

- Understand an early intervention team's function and composition as described in Part H of the Individuals with Disabilities Education Act (IDEA) of 1990, PL 101-476
- Understand that parents are members of the early intervention team and are the primary decision makers for their families
- Become familiar with three different models of teaming, recognize the functions of team members within each model, and understand how each model supports parent membership
- Understand the advantages and disadvantages of each model of teaming
- Recognize other factors that affect early intervention teams   ◆

> *"The purpose of a team is to share the work, the*
> *inspiration, the camaraderie, and the success of the task at hand."*

> —Failey (1993, p. 33)

The individualized family service plan (IFSP) is the heart of early intervention. The team is the mechanism that makes the heart (i.e., the IFSP process) work. In early intervention, the team approach recognizes that young children with disabilities typically have multifaceted needs that can be addressed more effectively by a team than by a single service provider. Effective teamwork can result in integrated and coordinated services for young children and their families. It also can be very satisfying to the people who provide those services.

A team is a group of people with a common goal who work together to make decisions and find solutions to problems related to shared tasks (Bruder & Bologna, 1993; Bruder, Lippman, Bologna, & Derrickson, 1991; Kilgo, Clarke, & Cox, 1990; Rossetti, 1991; Scholtes, 1988). Early intervention team members share common tasks, including conducting evaluations and assessments of the child, identifying and gaining access to resources, and planning and providing intervention services. They also face common challenges, such as establishing a shared vision and philosophy and learning how to work together well to make decisions, solve problems, and carry out their responsibilities.

The early intervention team is guided by the family and is responsible for making collaborative decisions to meet the needs of both the family and their child who is eligible for birth-to-3 services. A team is formed for each family and includes service providers from at least two professional disciplines. Parents are full members of the team and can include any support person they would like on the team. The early intervention team typically comprises individuals from more than one agency and provides services in a variety of natural environments for the child and family. According to the Individuals with Disabilities Education Act Amendments of 1991, PL 102-119, a family may deal with one or more teams, and a service provider may participate on many different teams. These are some of the unique features that characterize the early intervention team, and they will influence the functioning of each family's team.

This chapter outlines the major responsibilities of an early intervention team as defined by Part H of IDEA, including the role of the family on the team. In addition, three models of teaming used commonly in early intervention—multidisciplinary, interdisciplinary, and transdisciplinary—are described, and advantages and disadvantages of each are examined. Other factors that affect a team, such as variability in team members' agencies and leadership styles, are also discussed.

THE HALLMAN STORY

Kyle Hallman has received services from an early intervention program since he was 15 months old for delays in motor and communication development and differences in his social interaction skills. At 26 months, Kyle has just experienced major developmental growth. A respiratory problem that frequently left him sick and often too tired or uncomfortable to concentrate on developmental tasks was recently identified and treated. It took seven visits to physicians and nurses in specialty clinics over the course of 2 months to diagnose the problem. His parents, Sharon and Bill, and the service providers on their birth-to-3 team finally are seeing the benefits. Kyle's energy is more focused, and he interacts more with his family and with the service providers who work with him in various settings. He is exhibiting new skills and, most importantly, new curiosities and desires. Various team members, including his parents, have been talking about these new milestones with a number of service providers, all of whom collected their information separately. It has occurred to Sharon and Bill that it would be a good idea to assemble the various people who work with their family to discuss Kyle's latest medical findings and developmental gains and how these relate to members' work with Kyle.

Kyle receives the majority of his early intervention services from the local birth-to-3 program. The services are provided in his home or at the home of his child care provider. In addition, Kyle receives private therapy services periodically. Because of the diversity of team members, they do not see Kyle at the same time or place. Members cannot rely on casual encounters to meet with one another. Instead, they must maintain communication by exchanging notes, making telephone calls, and scheduling meetings.

Sharon and Bill have asked Nola, their service coordinator, to help them gather the team together: the service providers from the birth-to-3 program (an educator, a motor specialist, and a speech-language pathologist), their family child care provider, and the occupational therapist and the speech-language pathologist who see Kyle occasionally. They also invited Sharon's sister, Beverly, who spends considerable time with the family. The Hallmans wanted to update the team regarding Kyle's medical information; learn more about the gains seen by others; and share their observations, concerns, and priorities about next steps. They asked for an IFSP review and revision.

Together with Nola, Sharon and Bill picked the offices of the private therapists as the place for the meeting, worked out an agenda, and made telephone calls to invite the team. Sharon also decided that she would lead the meeting. In making the calls to invite people to the meeting, one of the staff from the birth-to-3 program questioned Sharon about why they were not meeting at the office of the birth-to-3 program; she expressed concerns about traveling elsewhere. Sharon was upset as a result of the conversation and had second thoughts about leading the meeting. With Nola's support, however, she stuck to her decisions but felt a little nervous about what would happen.

Sharon did lead the meeting, giving her update and asking team members for their ideas. She and Bill asked that someone take notes because they were worried that they might not remember everything. At first there was some tension among a few of the people at the meeting. Sharon had not realized that some people did not know one another very well. As the meeting progressed and attention focused on Kyle's needs, however, information and ideas were exchanged freely among team members. Sharon and Bill asked that new outcomes for the IFSP be rewritten during a future meeting of Sharon, Bill, and the service coordinator. The Hallmans guided the team by asking for members' observations and ideas and by seeking group consensus concerning Kyle's intervention services. At the meeting's end, several people approached Sharon and Bill to tell them how helpful the meeting had been. When Sharon was talking to a friend a couple of days later, her friend commented on how assertive Sharon had been in organizing the meeting and playing a leadership role. Sharon responded, "I can't imagine it any other way."

THE EARLY INTERVENTION TEAM AS DEFINED BY PART H OF IDEA

Political issues, economic conditions, and cultural trends affect an early intervention team even when members are unaware of their impact. Federal, state, and local laws and regulations also influence a team. Paying attention to the context in which these factors operate can increase a team's effectiveness, reduce stress for team members, and enhance services for the child and family. An important part of the context in early intervention is Part H of IDEA. This section discusses the provisions of Part H as they relate to early intervention teams.

The family-centered early intervention team consists of a child's parents and all of the people who provide formal and informal supports to the family. They are united by the common goal of supporting and strengthening the family in relation to the development of their child with disabilities. According to Part H of IDEA, the provision of integrated and coordinated early intervention services is the responsibility of a multidisciplinary team comprising the child's parents and service providers from two or more fields. Primary functions for service providers on the team include the following:

- Providing multidisciplinary evaluations and assessments
- Participating in the development of the IFSP
- Supporting family members as primary decision makers

Team members may also take part in other tasks relevant to Part H of IDEA, such as implementing and evaluating the IFSP; identifying and gaining access to services; participating in public awareness activities; helping with program development, implementation, and evaluation; and participating in staff development activities.

Part H of IDEA identifies the early intervention services supported by the law, sets standards for who can provide those services, specifies that services be provided in natural environments, and establishes the parents as members of the early intervention team. Mandates set the parameters for who participates on the early intervention team, what disciplines and agencies or programs are represented, and in which environments services are provided. Nevertheless, each family's team will respond differently to the unique needs of the child and family.

ACTIVITY: *The Hallmans' Early Intervention Team*

◆ ◆ ◆   The Hallman story shows one configuration of an early intervention team. Before proceeding with this chapter, return to the story and answer these questions about the Hallmans' early intervention team:

1. What early intervention services do the Hallmans receive?
2. Who is on the Hallmans' early intervention team?
3. What programs or agencies do the team members represent?
4. In which environments are services provided? ◆

Early Intervention Services Mandated by Part H of IDEA

A variety of services specified in the Individuals with Disabilities Education Act Amendments comprises the core of fundable services within the early intervention system, including family training, counseling and home visits, speech pathology and audiology, occupational therapy, physical therapy, psychological services, assistive technology devices and services, service coordination, medical services (as necessary for diagnostic and evaluation services), early identification, screening and assessment, related health services (as necessary to enable the infant or toddler to benefit from early intervention services), vision services, and transportation. Particular services can be provided to a child and family by early intervention team members who are qualified to perform those services. States' interpretations of early intervention services and the addition of three services (i.e., assistive technology devices and services, vision services, and transportation) with the reauthorization of Part H of PL 102-119 indicate that the list of services is still evolving.

Although this list limits the services that can be funded under the law, an individual family may utilize other formal or informal support services to assist them in meeting their family's or child's needs. Other services could include support from a religious group, well-child medical care, carpentry services to make a home accessible, or any service or resource that would facilitate achievement of a child's and family's outcomes.

Who Is on the Team?

As mentioned previously, Part H specifies that the early intervention team comprise the child's parents and service providers from two or more disciplines. There is a range of service providers upon which to draw, including professionals from the core disciplines outlined in Part H as well as other professionals and people in a family's formal and informal support network. The core disciplines are the following:

*   Audiology
*   Early childhood special education

- Family therapy
- Nursing
- Nutrition
- Occupational therapy
- Orientation and mobility
- Pediatrics and other branches of medicine
- Physical therapy
- Psychology
- Social work
- Speech-language pathology

Several of the core disciplines include a continuum of professional positions. Physical therapy includes physical therapists and physical therapist assistants; occupational therapy includes registered occupational therapists and certified occupational therapy assistants; nutrition includes registered nutritionists and dietitian technicians; education includes certified teachers and educational assistants or paraeducators; and nursing includes registered nurses and licensed practical nurses. Some of these positions permit greater independence than others. For example, service providers at the assistant level (i.e., certified occupational therapy assistant, dietitian technician, physical therapist assistant) require supervision from a professional in their discipline to carry out their responsibilities (Pickett, 1995). Team composition varies and depends on the needs of the child and preferences of the family. The following sections examine more closely the potential composition of the early intervention team.

Personnel Standards on the Early Intervention Team

The law specifies the personnel who may provide early intervention services. States are responsible for establishing personnel standards within their early intervention systems that meet the highest state requirements for each discipline. Standards vary from state to state and depend on past practice, current licensing practices of individual disciplines, and the skills required for early intervention. For example, although one state may require a Bachelor of Science (B.S.) degree in nursing, another might require a Master of Science (M.S.) degree or a registered nurse (R.N.) license. With regard to speech-language pathology, it is likely that the master's degree is the standard requirement in most states. The overall purpose of establishing standards is to ensure a family that qualified personnel will be available to provide services for their child.

Parent Positions on the Early Intervention Team

As states defined team composition for their early intervention service systems, many looked beyond the list of core disciplines. A growing number of states, including Wisconsin, Illinois, Hawaii, Massachusetts, and North

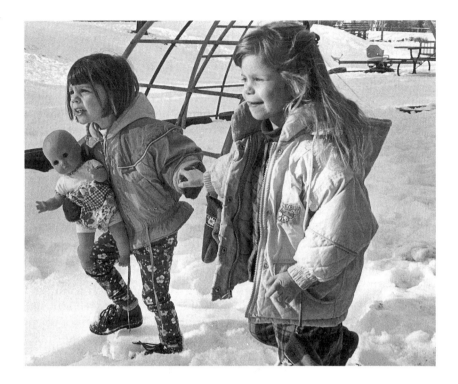

Carolina, to name a few, have created parental positions to recognize the significance of what parents have to offer to one another (Striffler, 1993).

For example, Wisconsin includes *parent facilitators* in its list of qualified personnel. Parent facilitators' responsibilities could include providing information and support to families, establishing parent-to-parent support networks, coordinating services, and participating in program planning and policy development. Hawaii has a project in which *parent involvement specialists* are hired to provide ongoing service coordination to families and to assist families in developing and implementing their IFSPs. The project also identifies *parent involvement assistants* who carry out these same responsibilities under the supervision of social workers or educators (Striffler, 1993).

Other Key Members of the Early Intervention Team

States are also looking for other ways to expand the number of qualified personnel who can provide early intervention services. This is being done through the development of significant roles for other personnel on the team. Some states are utilizing and training non–discipline-specific service providers and service providers without bachelor's degrees to carry out various aspects of early intervention.

For example, Massachusetts has recognized the importance of employing personnel who understand and are sensitive to the culture of a community. The state's personnel model includes a *community outreach worker* position. The position requires an individual to "have experience and knowledge of the community and its resources, and experience or training in the designated role" (Striffler, 1993, p. 11). Other states, such as Illinois, Maine, Texas, South Carolina, and Utah, have created positions for aides, assistants, and/or associates. These personnel provide supportive early intervention services in a variety of settings to enhance available services (Striffler, 1993). In all instances, service providers 1) carry out intervention strategies developed and monitored by professionals, and 2) provide general support services with supervision. This arrangement can be mutually beneficial for all involved: supervising professionals, supervised professionals, and families. Supervisors increase the range of services they can provide, the supervised professional has a meaningful role on the early intervention team, and families receive services from a range of qualified personnel.

Other members on the early intervention team are those identified by the family. For some this may be an early childhood educator or the family's child care provider. Although not mentioned specifically in the law, their roles are becoming increasingly important as services are provided in natural environments. Grandparents, friends, and other advocates identified by the family may be members of the family's early intervention team. These members, like the other team members, support the family in identifying and receiving the supports necessary to meet outcomes.

Team Members' Agencies

A family's early intervention team may include service providers from a single agency. Often, however, the team includes service providers from several different agencies to address the child's and family's comprehensive needs adequately. A host of agencies could potentially employ the team members who provide the broad array of early intervention services available through Part H. Part H establishes an interagency program in which each state identifies a lead agency, such as health, education, or social services. The numbers and types of agencies in a community are largely influenced by the state's lead agency and how the state's service system is organized. Members of an early intervention team can come from a variety of places, for example, county agencies, private or nonprofit agencies, public or private clinics, hospitals, social services agencies, or schools, just to name a few.

This interagency structure adds another dimension to the configuration of an early intervention team. Teams in which all or most members are employed by a single agency will likely have interaction styles that differ from those of teams whose members represent two or more agencies. Consider what happened to the Hallmans' team when members from different agencies gathered for a meeting. At first there was tension among the team members from different agencies. As the conversation focused on the team's common goal of supporting Kyle, however, the tension decreased.

In summary, a family's team could include any of the people described earlier. They may be employed by a single agency or by several different agencies. According to Part H, the only given is that the team include the family and representatives from at least two disciplines. Getting to know who is on the team, what each member does, who is responsible for what, and something about each member's agency are important aspects of teaming in early intervention.

Natural Environments for Early Intervention Services

Part H further delineates early intervention by requiring that services be provided in natural environments. Part H stipulates that

> To the maximum extent appropriate, infants and toddlers must be provided early intervention services in natural environments, including the home, and community settings such as day care centers, in which children without disabilities participate. The term "natural environments" refers to settings that are natural or normal for age peers who have no apparent disability. (Individuals with Disabilities Education Act Amendments of 1991, 34 CFR 303, 12[b][1])

Often the primary natural environment for an infant or toddler is his or her own home. Other settings "normal for age peers who have no apparent disabilities" (34 CFR 303, 12[b][1]) could include group settings such as a neighborhood play group, a child care center, a community center, or even a story hour at the local public library.

A key question is, "What environments do the family identify as the most natural environments for their child?" The answer to this question helps determine the place at which the team delivers services as well as the nature of interactions among team members. For example, the interactions among team members who provide the majority of their services one at a time in a family's home will be very different from the interactions among members who are in a community program in which several staff are present at any given time. Where and when services are delivered determine how often and where team members cross paths. Do they call each other, see each other daily in their offices, pass in the halls of a child care center, or attend planned meetings?

The various natural settings in which a child may be served create logistical issues that a team must identify and address. For example, a team will have to determine where they will meet; this can be almost anywhere—homes, hospitals, clinics, child care centers, physicians' offices, or even over breakfast at McDonald's. A family-guided team meets at the location that is most suitable for the child's primary caregivers. Selecting locations for team meetings is an important team function that requires parents' input and guidance. In the Hallman story, Sharon and Bill decided they wanted to meet at the office of one of their son's private therapists, a place they visit periodically and where they feel comfortable and supported. Other options included the Hallman home, the home of the child care provider, and the office of the birth-to-3 program.

ACTIVITY: *The Hallman Story Revisited*

◆ ◆ ◆   Consider the information presented in this chapter about the range of personnel who can be on an early intervention team and the environments where services can be provided. Take another look at the Hallmans' early intervention team and consider your personal preferences.

1. If you were in Sharon's and Bill's place on the team, what changes might you want to make to the team? Would you want more or fewer people on the team? Why? Whom might you add or remove from the team?
2. If English were not your first language, whom might you add to the team? Why?
3. If Sharon were a single mother, would you want to make any changes in the team? If yes, what changes might you make? Why?
4. In what environments would you like to receive services? Why?   ◆

PARENTS AS TEAM MEMBERS AND DECISION MAKERS

"Families of children with disabilities have much to offer
a team, because we have so much to gain from the team."

—Failey (1993, p. 33)

Under the law, service providers have an obligation to facilitate parental participation on the early intervention team and to provide support and information so that family members can direct the team to the extent they prefer. Service providers are also responsible for ensuring that the service system is sensitive to the family's changing concerns and priorities. Thus, the early intervention team is dynamic, and parents' roles may alter depending on their circumstances.

Parents are full and essential members of the early intervention team. Service providers are members of the family's team (McGonigel & Garland, 1988; Nash, 1990). In practice, this means that parents may choose to lead the team in all activities or to share their roles with other team members, such as the service coordinator. Parents may participate as active decision makers, or they may take less active roles.

Parents' roles can change with time and circumstances. Parents may choose to be more active during a time of relative stability in their lives or when a transition is pending. During a health or personal crisis, parents may choose less active roles, looking for advice and guidance from service providers regarding decision making. Parents may choose many different roles as their child grows from a newborn to a toddler. There are no generalizations. Each family is unique and will choose their roles as they see fit (see Chapter 8). This is an important and central concept of Part H; to many service providers, it entails a conceptual shift in team organization and functioning:

> Families may not be eager to participate as team members initially. We need a "breaking in" period after learning of our child's disability, time to adjust to all the changes we must go through and all the emotions that accompany this. Time to learn the jargon and acronyms that we hear at every turn. When finally our anger and grief become determination and perseverance, we are able to make valuable contributions to the team effort. (Failey, 1993, p. 33)

The family's membership on the early intervention team opens doors to a system that is family guided to the extent that the family desires (Nash, 1990).

Supporting Parents as Full Members of the Early Intervention Team

Membership on an early intervention team whose other members are service providers is a new experience for some parents, just as having parents as full members on the team is new for some service providers. On the one hand, many people employed in early intervention have received at least some training and will continue to develop their skills as team members. Most parents, on the other hand, do not expect to be members of an early intervention team and find that the roles are thrust upon them as part of an unexpected series of events in their lives. This certainly was true for the Hallmans. McGonigel and Garland (1988) suggested that professionals should be less concerned with making a place for the family on the early intervention team and more concerned with developing strategies that will enable professionals to become members of the family's team.

Information Sharing

Sharing information is an essential strategy for supporting parents as guides of their teams. A number of studies (Able-Boone, 1993; Bailey, Buysse, Edmondson, & Smith, 1992; Brinckeroff & Vincent, 1986; Fallon & Harris, 1992) have shown that information is a key ingredient for having a high level of parent involvement in team activities, including decision making. Information is a powerful tool for comfortable and active involvement. The Hallmans felt comfortable organizing and leading their meeting primarily because they understood important information related to Kyle's development. They also believed that team members had valuable information and observations to contribute. They may not have always felt that way.

Service providers should be prepared to give parents whatever information they need to participate comfortably on the early intervention team. Parents may find information about the following to be helpful:

- The early intervention program, including procedural safeguards
- The child's development and service providers' impressions of his or her needs
- Current, complete, and accurate information about a child's particular disability, including ways to gain access to this information
- Service providers' ideas about outcomes for the child
- Differences in opinions among service providers on the team, if they occur
- Resources to meet the child's and family's needs and how to gain access to them
- The teaming process and ways in which the team can work together for the family

In all situations with families, it is important that assumptions are not made about what information a particular family wants or needs. It is always important to ask parents what information they would like to have and how they would like to receive it. Indeed, it was only after several conversations that the Hallmans understood what they wanted to gain from a team meeting. Like many families, the Hallmans may repeat the process with every new situation that comes up for Kyle. Talking and sharing written materials are the most common means of sharing information. Videotapes, audiotapes, photographs, drawings, or other forms of presentation can also be effective means of conveying a wealth of information relevant to early intervention.

Role Clarification

Service providers should also tell parents about the variety of roles parents may choose, including observer, active participant, or facilitator, among other roles. Because families come to early intervention programs with different experiences, it is important that assumptions not be made about what parents do or do not know about the teaming process. Many parents may never have participated on teams, read books about teams, or received training relevant to the teaming process; others may be professionals or businesspeople with much team experience.

Parents may need time to think about how they want to participate on the team. They may also want to be able to change their roles, or they may want information about what is required for the various roles. One courtesy noted by McGonigel, Johnson, and Kaufmann (1991), and used in the Hallman team meeting is to invite parents to be the initial speakers at team meetings. This gives them a chance to share their perspectives and to describe observations before service providers speak. If a parent is interested in being a facilitator, there are a variety of ways to support the parent in this role. One is for the parent to meet with other parents who have facilitated team activities for their children. Another is for the parent to outline facilitators' tasks with the service coordinator and to practice or role-play in advance of meetings. Videotaped examples can also be helpful in learning about various roles.

Common Vocabulary

Service providers also can facilitate parent participation by using language that is straightforward and free of jargon during conversations and in written documents (e.g., IFSPs, reports). Through training and experience, service providers often become fluent users of their disciplines' jargon. Specialized terminology has its uses, especially if everyone involved in a conversation shares a common vocabulary. On an early intervention team, which includes parents as well as people from several different disciplines, however, use of jargon can impede communication. During conversations as well as in written reports, team members should be careful to use commonly understood language whenever possible. And when technical terms must be used, they should be carefully explained.

Recognizing Family Needs

Family concerns will sometimes take precedence over team goals. For example, if a parent has not had enough sleep, is dealing with a medical emergency, or is facing a personal crisis involving a basic need such as food or housing, that parent will have concerns that take priority over those of the early intervention team. Sensitivity to the parent's needs and a caring response will go a long way toward supporting the parent as a team member.

ACTIVITY: *Supporting Families' Needs as Team Members*

◆ ◆ ◆   This section of the chapter has been devoted to parents' membership on their child's early intervention team. Consider the supports described previously in responding to the following questions:

1. What practices were used by the Hallmans?
2. What practices were not in place that could have enhanced the Hallmans' comfort with their primary roles in guiding their early intervention team? Consider Sharon and Bill separately.   ◆

MODELS OF TEAMING

Effective early intervention teams adopt a model of teaming that will assist members in accomplishing their shared tasks. A model offers a structure that focuses on team-identified outcomes related to the provision of quality services for young children and their families. The model often is a unique combination of several approaches that match a team's vision and goals (Bruder & Bologna, 1993). Knowing the characteristics of the various team models and the advantages and disadvantages of each can help early intervention service providers understand their own teams and communicate with families about how their teams are organized. Such information can also help teams make decisions about directions for their continued development.

Characteristics of Three Team Models

Early intervention teams are typically organized according to one of three models of teaming—multidisciplinary, interdisciplinary, or transdisciplinary—or a combination of these. Each model has its own structure for interactions among team members. The three models differ in their approaches to initial contact with families, evaluation and assessment, IFSP development and monitoring, and implementation of service plans. Factors such as guiding philosophy and vision, channels of communication, time commitments for the teaming process, team member responsibilities, and leadership influence which model a team selects and how services will be delivered within that model (Bruder & Bologna, 1993; Woodruff & McGonigel, 1988).

A team that values frequent, ongoing communication and group problem solving and decision making may choose one model, whereas a team whose members want to work more independently may use a different model. Other contributing factors, such as the locations of team members and the environments in which services are delivered, also affect a team's decision about which model to use. A team whose members are employed primarily by one agency may choose a different model than would a team whose members work out of multiple agencies. Similarly, channels of communication among team members who provide home-based services would differ from those used by people who work primarily in a center.

Parent involvement is another important variable. Some models are more conducive to parent membership than others, although all models can be adapted for the full involvement of parents. Regardless of which model or combination of models a team uses, the dynamics of interactions among members will vary, and there are advantages and disadvantages to each approach.

Multidisciplinary Teams

On multidisciplinary teams, members share common goals but work independently of one another to represent their own disciplines. Although members may be aware of one another's activities and may share resources, an overall group effort is not required. There may be communication among members, but it is not built into the model. Team members usually function separately, with little integration across fields. Each member is usually trained in a particular discipline and therefore uses discipline-specific skills. A discipline's roles and responsibilities are understood and respected. Typically, each member of the team conducts an evaluation relevant to his or her discipline and then develops and implements a service plan related to that discipline (Bruder & Bologna, 1993; Council for Exceptional Children, 1988; McGonigel & Garland, 1988; Rossetti, 1991; Woodruff & McGonigel, 1988).

For example, given this model, a social worker would conduct a family-directed assessment, a physical therapist would evaluate and treat a child's motor problems, and a speech-language pathologist would address communication issues. Peterson (1987) compared multidisciplinary teams to *parallel play* in young children: "side by side, but separate." Parents typically meet individually with each team member and often receive information related to a specific area of development. Parents also may be invited to share information.

Interdisciplinary Teams

Members of interdisciplinary teams also share common goals. However, these teams have a commitment to communication among team members, including families. They have formal lines of communication to encourage interactions regarding evaluations and assessments, planning, and intervention. Typically, team members perform tasks separately and then come together at scheduled times to share information, develop plans, and solve problems. Generally, each member is responsible for tasks related directly to his or her discipline (Bruder & Bologna, 1993; Council for Exceptional Children, 1988; McGonigel & Garland, 1988; Rossetti, 1991; Woodruff & McGonigel, 1988). Because there are formal channels of communication among members, staff from different disciplines have opportunities to learn from one another. For example, an early childhood special education teacher and an occupational therapist would have numerous opportunities to learn about the other's work, each recognizing their overlapping interests as well as the unique knowledge and skills that each brings to the team. For instance, they might learn that they are both interested in play. The occupational therapist might learn more about creating learning environments, and the early childhood special education teacher might learn more about feeding skills. The learning opportunities are incidental and are based on shared experiences. No formal system for the transfer of skills is involved. Fixed times for communication among members (e.g., at IFSP meetings) ensure that parents have at least some opportunity to share and receive information about their child.

Transdisciplinary Teams

Transdisciplinary teams use a systematic process for sharing roles and crossing disciplinary boundaries to maximize communication, interaction, and cooperation among members (Bruder & Bologna, 1993; Council for Exceptional Children, 1988; McGonigel & Garland, 1988; Rossetti, 1991; Woodruff & McGonigel, 1988). Team members make a commitment to teach, learn, and work together across disciplinary boundaries to implement coordinated services. Typically, decisions are made by consensus, and family participation is crucial. Parents are full, active team members and can coordinate services if they so choose.

Role release is an essential component of transdisciplinary teaming. Service providers using this model assume the roles of professionals in their own and other fields. This is not because certain fields are not represented. Rather, it is because team members believe that intervention is more effective when they share knowledge and skills. Teaching discipline-specific skills to others and learning new skills from other disciplines involve several separate but related stages (Woodruff & McGonigel, 1988). These stages are described in Table 5.1. To ensure that families receive services from qualified personnel, it is essential that transdisciplinary team members complete an appropriate training process resulting in role release.

On a transdisciplinary team, members from the various disciplines may carry out an *arena assessment* to gather important planning information (Orelove & Sobsey, 1991; Woodruff & McGonigel, 1988). In an arena assessment, one team member usually is responsible for interacting directly with the child as another team member supports the family. Team members from a variety of disciplines then observe and record the child's behaviors. The developmental areas observed by each team member are agreed upon in advance of the assessment, and each member's

Table 5.1.   Stages of transdisciplinary skills development

Role extension	Team members carry out self-directed study in their own disciplines or areas of specialty.
Role enrichment	The discipline specialists are well versed in their own areas of specialty but have increased awareness and understanding of other disciplines gained through defined terminology and shared information about practices.
Role expansion	Team members exchange ideas and information about how to make knowledgeable observations and program recommendations outside of their own areas of specialty.
Role exchange	With backgrounds in theory, methods, and procedures from other disciplines, team members implement techniques from those disciplines. (This is best accomplished with team members working side by side.)
Role release	Team members practice new techniques from other disciplines under the supervision of the discipline specialists, who are accountable for those techniques.
Role support	The discipline specialists provide support to team members as they carry out discipline-specific interventions.

Adapted from Orelove and Sobsey (1991) and Woodruff and McGonigel (1988).

observations often (but not always) relate directly to their disciplines. One service provider may observe cognitive skills while others observe motor skills, communication skills, and/or social interactions. The person interacting with the child could be one of the child's parents or siblings, or a provider from a specific discipline closely related to the child's needs. This person can be the same person or different people as needed throughout the assessment. The important aspect is to communicate about 1) who will do what and when; and 2) how the plan will change, if needed, to meet the needs of the child and family. The observers can request that the person interacting with the child try certain activities that may enable the child to demonstrate certain skills; the person supporting the parent(s) can gather information for other team members.

The arena assessment is one way in which transdisciplinary team members can work together to share information and tasks and reduce redundancy for children and families. Providing integrated services with one team member serving as the primary service provider receiving support from the rest of the team is another way. In such situations, for example, a speech-language pathologist may be the primary service provider for the family. He or she would work in all areas of development and would receive consultation and role support from other team members (e.g., parents, teachers, physical therapists).

The Combination Model

In reality, many teams decide to combine elements of one or more of the models described here. A variety of factors might influence such a decision. In many instances, the combination model might be the most practical way to maximize available resources to meet the needs of a child and his or her family. A highly specialized multidisciplinary team may facilitate communication among team members and open up possibilities for increased parent involvement.

For example, on a given interagency team there may be a core of primary service providers, such as therapists or teachers, who favor the transdisciplinary model. Other members of the same team who have less frequent or more specialized contact with families may favor either the multidisciplinary or the interdisciplinary model. Nevertheless, whether issues involve location, staff skills, or communication channels, any team model can be adapted to fit the needs of individual families and communities.

ACTIVITY: *The Hallman Team Model*

◆ ◆ ◆   Picture the Hallmans' team. Think about the disciplinary roles and boundaries of the members, the channels of communication, and the parents' levels of participation:

1. What model of teaming do you think the Hallmans' team used?
2. What led you to that conclusion?
3. What were the advantages and disadvantages of this model for the family and staff?
4. If the team had been using another model, how might the story have changed? ◆

Advantages and Disadvantages of Teaming Models

Each model has advantages and disadvantages. The transdisciplinary model integrates principles of coordinated and family-centered services to a greater extent than do the others. It includes parents as team members in planning and decision making, and its structure facilitates greater coordination, communication, and sharing among team members. The transdisciplinary model is most conducive to a holistic approach that views the child as a whole person and a member of the family system. This model recognizes commonalities among disciplines, such as knowledge of child development or family systems theory, as well as specialized practices within each discipline. Members of transdisciplinary teams have experience in listening and learning from others as well as in transferring their skills to others. These skills are essential for supporting a family. They are also important for supporting service providers and other members of a family's informal support network.

One advantage of both multidisciplinary and interdisciplinary teams is that their members are likely to be highly skilled in their specialty areas. Either of these models would be more practical than the transdisciplinary model when team members come from more than one agency.

The major disadvantages of the multidisciplinary team are 1) the lack of communication among members; 2) the emphasis on looking only at one particular aspect of the child; and 3) the possibility for duplication of services, especially with a young child. The child may not be seen as a whole person or as a member of the family system, and services may be fragmented as a result. Families have frequently told stories about the number of times they have had to tell the same story to different people, about duplications of services such as evaluation and assessment, and about the mixed messages they have received from different service providers.

The interdisciplinary and transdisciplinary models avoid these pitfalls by increasing parent involvement, communication among members, and coordination of services. In the interdisciplinary model, the primary complication is related to "turf" issues. Specialists maintain their disciplinary roles and must "sort out" the overlap. For example, nurses, dietitians, occupational therapists, and speech-language pathologists all have expertise with problems associated with feeding. On an interdisciplinary team, people from these four professions must agree on a division of re-sponsibilities. In the process of sorting out roles and solving problems, members of an interdisciplinary team have opportunities to learn from one another and expand their knowledge bases about other areas.

A transdisciplinary team approaches roles and responsibilities from a different perspective. In deciding who will do what, team members con-sider the parents' preferences, the size of the team, the experience of team members, the family's primary contacts, and the compatibility of schedules. If a child has multiple needs and the family prefers to have fewer service providers involved, members of a transdisciplinary team can accommodate the family's preference and still meet the child's devel-opmental needs. One or two team members who practice *role exchange* and *role support* (see Table 5.1) would be prepared to address the family's multifaceted needs. A multidisciplinary or interdisciplinary team whose members use discipline-specific skills, however, would be challenged by this family's preference. They might not feel comfortable supporting the family and meeting the child's feeding, mobility, play, and communica-tion needs without including an occupational therapist, a physical thera-pist, a teacher, a nurse, a social worker, and/or a speech-language pathol-ogist on the team.

Transdisciplinary teaming requires a commitment of time from team members, their supervisors, and agency administrators. It requires a will-ingness to teach, learn, and work across traditional disciplinary bound-aries. It assumes a transfer of learning in the context of practical applica-tions. If members come from more than one agency, considerable work is required to organize time and to keep channels of communication open.

Laws designed to protect people place limitations on role release by some disciplines such as nursing and medicine. The major risk of the transdisciplinary model is that practitioners may believe they have ac-quired skills in areas outside of their own disciplines when, in fact, they have not taken all the necessary steps toward role release. Indeed, there may be times when a child's or family's needs warrant the direct exper-tise of a highly trained specialist.

On all teams, regardless of which teaming model(s) is used, strengths should be emphasized and obstacles addressed. A team's model should provide a structure for addressing the common goals of early intervention in providing comprehensive and family-centered services. In keeping with the spirit of Part H of IDEA, a team's model should accommodate parents' preferences for participation and recognize that these preferences may change over time. On multidisciplinary and interdisciplinary teams, open communication can be facilitated and parent involvement in-creased. On a transdisciplinary team, people with greater expertise can be brought onto the team as needed. Drawing upon the best of what each model has to offer gives an early intervention team the most flexibility in meeting a family's needs and increasing participants' satisfaction.

ACTIVITY: *Creating a Product*

◆ ◆ ◆ One way to get a feel for the differences among the models of teaming is to participate in the training activity described by Beninghof and Singer (1992). In this activity, three groups are asked to make something with a variety of arts and crafts materials. Each group is given separate instructions, but all the groups have the common goals of making something, having fun, and sharing their finished products with the other groups.

Members of the first group are to work individually in isolation from others. They are not to talk with or watch others. They may not share materials, and they are not to combine their individual products to make a final product. Members of the second group are allowed to talk to one another, but they cannot share materials. They are to combine their individual products at the end of the activity to make one final product. Members of the third group are to work together to make a product. They are to share materials, talk, and agree on the product that is made.

After completing the activity, consider the following questions:

1. Can you guess which group follows the multidisciplinary model? The interdisciplinary model? The transdisciplinary model?
2. What do you see as the advantages and disadvantages of each group? Think about the processes and products.
3. Which group would be most conducive to full parent involvement? ◆

Other Factors that Affect a Team's Model of Teaming

There are a number of other factors that a team may want to consider before deciding which model or models of teaming to utilize. Since the passage of Part H, the context for practices in early intervention has changed. Service providers have new systems in which to work, new skills to learn, and new roles to play. Many agencies are restructuring their early intervention programs in response to Part H. Choosing a new model or changing an old model of teaming may be part of these restructurings. Understanding the advantages and disadvantages of each model and considering other issues, such as training of personnel, interagency teams, leadership, and roles of team members, can help team members to choose the best model of teaming for their particular circumstances. The following sections highlight several areas of changing practices that may affect teams' organizations and structures.

Training of Personnel

Many early intervention service providers receive training exclusively in their areas of specialty. This training focuses primarily on discipline-specific knowledge and skills and offers few opportunities to learn about the skills and practices of other disciplines. In addition, few early intervention service providers receive training in teaching their skills to others, understanding organizational systems, and/or assuming leadership roles. These are all important skills for achieving the goals of early intervention. No team can operate effectively if members work in complete isolation from one another (Mariano, 1989; McGonigel & Garland, 1988). Therefore, many current service providers need to learn new skills in order to be effective team members.

Interagency Teams

Interagency teams can offer an increased array of services and expertise to families and children. Kyle's team, for example, includes staff from a birth-to-3 program, therapists from a private clinic, and a family child care provider, as well as a multitude of physicians who see Kyle routinely. In some communities, health care providers and an interagency team may be the best or only way in which to address a combination of health care, social, and educational needs. In addition, an interagency team can be more flexible in responding to a family's preferences. For example, a child who would otherwise need to travel to a regional hospital for physical therapy might be seen at a neighborhood clinic as a result of an interagency team effort.

Service providers must understand not only the workings of the teams within the agencies that employ them but also the functions of teams in agencies with which they collaborate. For example, to ease the tensions among members of the Hallmans' team, it would be well worth their time to learn about the practices of other members' agencies. For instance, the occupational therapist might want to know which model of teaming the birth-to-3 program uses, how staff make decisions, what leadership styles and channels of communication are used by the team within the program, and who the key contact people are. Staff from the birth-to-3 program might want to know similar aspects about the therapist's situation. The following are some questions that may help teams from different agencies as they begin to work together:

- Who will be on the interagency team?
- What will be the mission and goals of the interagency team?
- What's the expertise/specialty of the team?
- Which model of teaming will be used?
- Who will lead the interagency team?
- How will parents be included on the interagency team?
- Who will be the primary contact(s)?
- When will the team meet?
- When are the best times to call?
- How will decisions be made and problems solved?

When engaging in interagency teaming, members should be well aware of the challenges involved in coordinating the activities of the team. Note the tensions among the members of the Hallmans' team. Maintaining a focus on the family can facilitate the team's efforts. (Chapter 7 of this book offers more suggestions for meeting the challenges of interagency teaming and collaboration.)

ACTIVITY: *Facilitating Communication*

◆ ◆ ◆   You are the occupational therapist working on the Hallmans' team, and you feel isolated from the rest of the team; however, you have a wonderful relationship with the family. You want to feel more involved with the ongoing activities of the team. You sensed some resistance on the part of the motor specialist from the birth-to-3 program when you talked with the Hallmans' service coordinator about team members having more frequent and ongoing communication with one another. Consider the following questions:

1. What do you see as the challenges and barriers to getting more involved?
2. Given these challenges and barriers, how would you go about getting more involved with the team? More specifically, what strategies could you use to facilitate communication among the members? What steps could you take to increase your involvement? ◆

Leadership

Teams need leadership to accomplish their goals. Yet, leadership styles are implied, not explicitly identified, in the three teaming models described. When choosing a teaming model, possible leadership styles also should be considered. Will the team have an authoritative decision maker who directs the team and makes all final decisions, or will leadership responsibilities rotate as the team seeks consensus in all matters (Rees, 1991; Rossetti, 1991)?

It is important to consider the implications of different leadership styles on the overall functioning of a team. Some styles are more conducive to parental involvement than others, and some provide more direction than others. For instance, a transdisciplinary team may favor a leadership style that empowers team members to participate in making only those decisions that affect them directly, or the team may seek group consensus before any decisions are made. Leadership responsibilities may also rotate on a transdisciplinary team. The primary service provider for the family may serve as the team's leader, or one of the parents may choose to lead the team.

Leadership on a multidisciplinary team may not be defined as clearly. There may be a single leader to whom all the different service providers report. Conversely, there may be no defined leader, and members may be responsible for making their own decisions in isolation.

On any interagency team, there may be several leaders, one from each member's agency, and they may or may not have compatible styles. Leadership styles may be built into all of the teaming models described here. The important things for team members to know are who a team's leader is; which type of leadership style is in operation; and what the implications of delivering comprehensive, family-centered early intervention services are.

Roles of Team Members

Early intervention service providers can assume many different roles. On each team, some members play primary roles, such as leadership roles, whereas others provide role support or consultation. In addition, if a team is assembled to meet the individual needs of the family, service providers may find that the roles they play vary from team to team. On one family's team, a service provider may be the service coordinator or a direct interventionist, while on another family's team, he or she may provide consultation for team members, supervise a program assistant, and/or support the family.

There are growing places for role support and consultation in early intervention. The transdisciplinary model of teaming addresses the issues of role support and consultation most directly because it has a series of training stages built into the teaming process. Members of teams using other teaming models can, however, engage in the process of learning how to transfer their skills and knowledge to others as well. As services increasingly are being provided in natural environments, it will be important for early intervention service providers to be adept at training others (Orelove & Sobsey, 1991). Yet, training will be a new activity for many early intervention service providers. For infants and toddlers to succeed in certain natural settings, such as in child care centers, preschools, and libraries, early intervention specialists (i.e., therapists and early childhood special education teachers) will want to support caregivers who have less specialized training. This will often mean balancing direct, hands-on service provision with the provision of skills training to other caregivers. Transferring skills and knowledge to parents also is essential to fulfill the spirit and mandates of Part H.

SUMMARY

This chapter highlights the importance of teaming in early intervention. A team approach is mandated by legislation that sets parameters for what services early intervention teams can provide, who can provide those services, and in which environments team members can work. The legislation also establishes the spirit of the early intervention team. Parents are full members of their teams and have options and flexibility regarding their levels of involvement. Throughout this chapter, the importance of having parents on early intervention teams is stressed, and examples illustrate how parent involvement can be achieved.

Models of teaming and their respective advantages and disadvantages are also described. Adapting models to build on strengths, overcome obstacles, and meet needs in a variety of situations was stressed. All teams need skilled and experienced personnel, strong channels of communication among members, leadership, and parent involvement.

The next chapter addresses team dynamics in more detail. The skills discussed will help early intervention team members to 1) increase their understandings of the dynamics of their teams, and 2) build skills to facilitate increased, positive interactions with other team members. These are essential skills for all teams regardless of the teaming model that is used.

DISCUSSION QUESTIONS

◆ ◆ ◆
1. What are the major responsibilities of an early intervention team? Which is the most important in your opinion?
2. Which models of teaming were used by a team of which you have been a part? Were all the members from the same program or agency? How were parents included on the team?
3. What are the variables that a newly formed early intervention team would want to consider before deciding on a model of teaming? Cite three reasons for your choices.
4. Imagine that you work or are about to work for an early intervention agency that has used the multidisciplinary teaming model for many years. You know of the transdisciplinary model through your training, and you would like to try it. How could you encourage your agency to try it? What additional training might agency staff need to make such a change?   ◆

REFERENCES

Able-Boone, H. (1993). Family participation in the IFSP process: Family or professional driven. *Infant–Toddler Intervention: The Transdisciplinary Journal, 3*(1), 63–71.

Bailey, D., Buysse, V., Edmondson, R., & Smith, T. (1992). Creating family-centered services in early intervention: Perceptions of professionals in four states. *Exceptional Children, 58*(4), 298–305.

Beninghof, A.M., & Singer, A.L. (1992). Transdisciplinary teaming: An inservice training activity. *Teaching Exceptional Children, 24*(4), 70–73.

Brinckeroff, J., & Vincent, L. (1986). Increasing parental decision-making at the individual education program meeting. *Journal of the Division for Early Childhood, 11*, 46–58.

Bruder, M.B., & Bologna, T. (1993). Collaboration and service coordination for effective early intervention. In W. Brown, S.K. Thurman, & L.F. Pearl (Eds.), *Family-centered early intervention with infants and toddlers: Innovative cross-disciplinary approaches* (pp. 103–127). Baltimore: Paul H. Brookes Publishing Co.

Bruder, M.B., Lippman, C., Bologna, T., & Derrickson, J. (1991). *Higher education faculty training institute manual.* New York: New York Medical College, Mental Retardation Institute.

Council for Exceptional Children. (1988). *Early intervention for infants and toddlers: A team effort (Eric Digest* No. 461). Reston, VA: Author.

Failey, R.S. (1993). Parental perspectives. In K.F. Steckol (Ed.), *Teams and teamwork* (p. 33). Rockville, MD: American Speech-Language-Hearing Association.

Fallon, M.A., & Harris, M.B. (1992). Encouraging parent participation in early intervention programs. *Infant–Toddler Intervention: The Transdisciplinary Journal, 2*(2), 141–146.

Individuals with Disabilities Education Act (IDEA) of 1990, PL 101-476. (October 30, 1990). Title 20, U.S.C. 1400 et seq: *U.S. Statutes at Large, 104,* 1103–1151.

Individuals with Disabilities Education Act Amendments of 1991, PL 102-119. (October 7, 1991). Title 20, U.S.C. 1400 et seq: *U.S. Statutes at Large, 105,* 587–608.

Kilgo, J.J., Clarke, B.A., & Cox, A. (Eds.). (1990). *Interdisciplinary infant and family services training: A professional training model.* Richmond: Virginia Institute for Developmental Disabilities.

Mariano, C. (1989). The case for interdisciplinary collaboration. *Nursing Outlook, 37*(6), 285–288.

McGonigel, M., & Garland, C. (1988). The individualized family service plan and the early intervention team: Team and family issues and recommended practices. *Infants and Young Children, 1*(1), 10–21.

McGonigel, M.J., Johnson, B.H., & Kaufmann, R.K. (Eds.). (1991). *Guidelines and recommended practices for the individualized family service plan* (2nd ed.). Bethesda, MD: Association for the Care of Children's Health.

Nash, J.K. (1990). Public Law 99-457: Facilitating family participation on the multidisciplinary team. *Journal of Early Intervention, 14*(4), 318–326.

Orelove, F.P., & Sobsey, D. (1991). *Educating children with multiple disabilities: A transdisciplinary approach* (2nd ed.). Baltimore: Paul H. Brookes Publishing Co.

Peterson, N. (1987). *Early intervention for handicapped and at risk children: An introduction to early childhood special education.* Denver: Love Publishing.

Pickett, A.L. (1995). Some thoughts on setting standards for the preparation of paraprofessionals. *New Directions, 16*(1 & 2), 1, 8.

Rees, F. (1991). *How to lead work teams: Facilitation skills.* San Diego: Pfeiffer & Co.

Rossetti, L.M. (1991). Models for infant–toddler assessment. In L.M. Rossetti (Ed.), *Infant–toddler assessment* (pp. 55–86). San Diego: College Hill.

Scholtes, P.R. (1988). *The team handbook: How to use teams to improve quality.* Madison, WI: Joiner Associates.

Striffler, N. (1993). *NEC*TAS synthesis report: Current trends in the use of paraprofessionals in early intervention and preschool services.* Chapel Hill, NC: National Early Childhood Technical Assistance System.

Woodruff, G., & McGonigel, M. (1988). Early intervention team approaches: The transdisciplinary model. In J. Gordon, P. Hutinger, M. Karnes, & J. Gallagher (Eds.), *Early childhood special education* (pp. 163–181). Reston, VA: Council for Exceptional Children

6

TEAM DYNAMICS AND COMMUNICATION

Linda I. Tuchman

◆◆◆

OBJECTIVES

◆ ◆ ◆ By completing this chapter, the reader will

- Understand the characteristics and dynamics of effective teams and the barriers to team functioning
- Recognize behaviors of team members that promote, as well as those that impede, team functioning
- Understand the implications of team dynamics for early intervention providers and parents
- Learn communication skills to enhance team processes
- Apply decision-making and conflict-management skills ◆

The early intervention team is the mechanism that carries out the functions of the individualized family service plan (IFSP) process, the heart of early intervention work. Like the human heart, the team is a complex and dynamic mechanism with many interrelated processes. The heart is one of the strongest muscles of the body, but it requires special care and maintenance to function at maximum capacity. Figuratively, it is sensitive and breaks easily, especially if not well understood. The early intervention team is also sensitive and requires careful attention to enable it to perform its role as a strong and vital mechanism in the early intervention process.

Because teams are common in the workplace, team dynamics and group process have been studied extensively. Early intervention teams can learn much from the literature about characteristics of effective teams, relationships among team variables, and dynamic processes such as leadership, communication, and problem solving that promote teamwork. Ancient wisdom—"two heads are better than one"—and modern management approaches both point toward teamwork as the preferred method for bringing people together to share knowledge and solve problems. This chapter discusses the characteristics and dynamics of successful teamwork, and emphasizes how these components can be used to enhance the effectiveness of the family-centered early intervention team.

THE ROLLINS STORY

It is 8:15 A.M. on Wednesday morning. Jacqui and Stuart Rollins are expected at the Seneca Early Intervention Program in 15 minutes for their 6-month IFSP review. On this particular morning, however, 8:30 is approaching all too soon for everyone involved.

Like many other times in the Rollinses' lives since their 18-month-old son, Joey, was born, things are not working out as planned. Jacqui and Stuart have been looking forward to meeting with staff from the Seneca Early Intervention Program. They have known some of the staff since Joey started receiving services at 3 months of age, and they feel they have a good, open relationship with members of Joey's team. The date of the review meeting was set well in advance so that Stuart could arrange time off from work. Stuart and Jacqui are not overly anxious about the meeting because of past, generally positive experiences at the early intervention center. However, they do have a few new questions they want to ask the team regarding a magazine article that Jacqui's aunt read concerning a new treatment for motor skill development in young children. They wonder if this would help Joey, especially since they are beginning to be concerned about his rate of progress.

By the time the Rollinses arrived at the meeting on Wednesday morning, they had nearly forgotten why they were there. The past few days had been terrible, topped off by another sleepless night. Joey had been sick for 3 days and hadn't had more than a few short periods of uninterrupted sleep during that time. Twice Tuesday night he awoke, stirring his whole family including his 3-year-old twin brothers, Toby and Jonathan, who sleep in the same room with him. The twins went back to sleep soon after Jacqui gave them some water and tucked them in again, but Joey had trouble falling back to sleep each time. Finally, he and Jacqui fell asleep in the early morning hours. Stuart had been up off and on all night with Jacqui's comings and goings.

When the alarm rang, no one in the Rollins household was eager to get up. Jacqui and Stuart had to force themselves out of bed. They had to get themselves ready, prepare for Jacqui's mother to come and take care of Joey, and get the twins ready to go to their child care provider's home. Luckily, Joey stayed asleep and they didn't have to wake him.

The Seneca staff expected the meeting to be congenial and fairly routine. They thought Joey was doing well, and they felt positive about their relationship with Jacqui (they had only met Stuart a few times, but each of those encounters had been positive). The staff did not make special preparations for the meeting. They assumed that Barbara Lander, the service coordinator, would facilitate the meeting and that it would be conducted like most other IFSP review meetings. Little did they know about the night the Rollinses had had or that they were stalled in a major traffic jam.

At 8:45 staff assembled for the meeting started to wonder where the Rollinses were. By 9:00 those with 9:45 appointments outside the center voiced concern that they wouldn't be able to stay much longer. Tensions started to mount as various ideas were put forth about what to do. Barbara called the Rollinses' house and learned they had left a few minutes late—but that did not explain why they had not arrived yet.

As Jacqui and Stuart entered the room, they suddenly felt completely overwhelmed. They became acutely aware of their exhaustion, frazzled nerves, and anxiety about the meeting. They also could not get a take on the mood in the room. Looking around the table, they got all kinds of messages about their late arrival. One person said, "I'm so glad you're here," while another abruptly announced he couldn't wait any longer. Others fidgeted with papers and were not sure what to do.

Stuart briefly apologized for being late and explained they had been stuck in traffic. Practically in the same breath, he asked their questions about the new treatment. No one at Seneca was prepared for that. The physical therapist, the most anxious to leave for his next appointment, gave an abrupt response about the treatment being unproven. Barbara tried to bring the meeting back to the IFSP review, but did not succeed. By now, all had joined in the conversation about the new treatment, giving various opinions. Tension was mounting. Jacqui felt bombarded with information, had difficulty focusing her attention, and became very quiet. Stuart sensed that his question was met with resistance and, being exhausted, reacted by asking more forceful questions. One staff member became defensive; nobody seemed to be listening to anyone. Finally the early intervention teacher suggested that they gather more information for the family to read about the treatment. What started out as a well-intended review meeting turned into a disaster for everyone. Barbara, as the service coordinator, decided to end the meeting and take time to talk with Jacqui and Stuart. The IFSP review meeting could wait. Dealing with their exhaustion and feelings could not.

TEAM DYNAMICS

Team building is a complex and dynamic process. Effective teams do not develop overnight, but build over time. Members need time to get to know each other, to understand their team's purpose, and to establish communication channels in order to develop trust. From trust flows creativity, flexibility, accomplishment, and satisfaction. Team members accustomed to working together become adept at understanding the dynamic processes of teamwork. They learn to identify and anticipate their own roles and those played by their colleagues. They anticipate the challenges and recognize the situational factors that affect their functioning. When team members understand the dynamics of the teaming process, members are more likely to get involved, and team effectiveness is enhanced.

However, the process is not easy and does not necessarily come naturally. Often in the building process, team members experience stress and discomfort as their team develops its identity and members establish modes of working together to meet common goals. Tensions can arise at the task and interpersonal levels. To achieve satisfactory outcomes, it is equally important for members to focus on the challenges of their interpersonal relationships as it is for them to emphasize the tasks the team is charged with accomplishing. The team provides a forum for addressing problems at both of these levels. Consider the dynamics of the Rollinses' situation that Wednesday morning: The team gathered for the task of reviewing Joey's IFSP and ended up dealing with the interpersonal tensions among team members.

The fluidity of the teaming process adds to the complexity of the early intervention team. Team composition is not static, and early intervention providers and parents often find themselves on more than one team, playing different roles on each. From day to day, as the needs of different children and families are addressed, the parent and interagency members of the team change. Staff turnover, common in early intervention programs, introduces further modifications in team composition. This variability heightens the importance of understanding team dynamics.

Characteristics of Effective Teams

Teams succeed because of the skills, commitment, and hard work of their members. Working on teams benefits the members who participate, and can have a positive effect on the quality of services provided. Although teams vary in structure (see Chapter 5), size, makeup, and numerous other variables, the literature cites qualities that are common to all effective teams.

Commitment to Mission and Time

Most descriptions of effective teams stress the importance of commitment to a common mission, purpose, and goals (e.g., Kilgo, Clarke, & Cox, 1990; Maddux, 1988; Quick, 1992; Scholtes, 1988; Spencer & Coye, 1988), as well as commitment of time so that the team can grow and develop to effectively accomplish its goals. The paramount goals of commitment to a common mission and of time are supported by a number of other processes that contribute to effective teams. Some of these qualities, frequently described in the literature, are highlighted in the paragraphs following.

Interdependence of Team Members

For teams to be successful, members must agree that they need each other to accomplish their goals. They must be willing to contribute and receive from the process; to share information, feelings, and responsibility for the team's work. In all teams, interdependence takes time to evolve and can take even longer in family-centered, interagency early intervention teams. Interdependence can be a great source of support for people who deal with complicated, and often emotionally difficult, situations. Often, interdependent team members develop a great deal of care for one another, their work, and the people they support. Without interdependence, team goals can often be sidetracked by competing priorities and tensions in interpersonal relations among team members.

Respect for Individual Differences

Although interdependence is essential, recognition of individual contributions and differences precedes interdependence. Effective teams are enriched by the diversity among their members. Members create a safe environment for exploring the differences among themselves; discussion of differences is encouraged, and divergent viewpoints are respected. Team members also recognize when problems occur from differences (e.g., values, beliefs, perspectives, actions) and are willing to grapple with the issues even though they know it may be difficult. They seek creative approaches to address friction or conflicts related to differences. They may not always find solutions to differences, but they often find ways to respect the differences among members. Team members frequently create their own language based on the common understandings engendered within the group.

Effective Use of Communication Skills Among Members

Communication is the foundation for interactions among team members and cuts across all aspects of team functioning. Members of effective teams value open communication and practice good communication skills to share ideas, make decisions, solve problems, support team members, and manage conflict. They also recognize that some types of communication, such as interrupting or changing the subject, can impede team progress. Communication skills are learned, with each individual responsible for his or her part of a communication interaction. Respectful listening is one of the most important basic communication skills. Time and again, parents tell professionals that "being heard" is essential to developing trusting relationships. When team members listen to each other they create an atmosphere that invites all members to participate and be heard.

Organizational Support and Sufficient Resources

Effective teams are supported by organizations that value their teams' work and provide sufficient time and resources for teams to accomplish their goals. Team members know their organization stands behind them and have then the confidence to proceed with their work. Supportive organizations recognize a team's accomplishments and accept mistakes as a normal part of teamwork. They also help teams gain access to appropriate resources. Without this support, there is a danger that team efforts will be meaningless. In early intervention, organizational support often comes from a variety of sources, and early intervention team members often devote substantial time to coordinating these diverse resources.

Leadership

In addition to organizational support, teams need effective leadership. All teams need a clearly defined leader, whether that individual is assigned, appointed, elected, or self-selected, and whether he or she serves permanently or rotates that responsibility among other team members. "Good leaders have vision, make good decisions, and share values with followers" (Mealy, 1984, p. 6). They understand their leadership style, and recognize their strengths and areas needing improvement. Effective leaders apply different skills under different circumstances. For example, an effective leader takes a strong position to direct a newly forming team or when conflict arises, but also knows when to take a lesser role to support team-directed activities. Some leaders have more decision-making authority than others; some may have the final say, whereas others depend on group consensus.

Leadership *roles* must also be clearly defined, even if varying over time. Members of early intervention teams are called upon to perform a variety of leadership functions such as giving guidance, facilitating meetings, making decisions, and securing resources for the team. Some service providers (e.g., Landerholm, 1990; Nash, 1990; Swan & Morgan, 1993) and parents have asserted that lack of clear leadership can be a problem for early intervention teams that meet in various configurations over time around individual families.

Defined Roles for Members

Clear roles and expectations contribute to the comfort and efficient functioning of team members. Thus, it is important for teams to clarify the roles and responsibilities of all team members, either by assigning roles, having members select roles or adhering to the roles of a particular position (e.g., speech-language pathologist assesses communication skills). Flexibility and clear communication concerning role boundaries are also valuable, especially in early intervention where the potential for overlapping responsibilities is great.

Team Participation in Decision Making

Effective teams give a voice to those who are involved in or affected by a decision. Typically this means that all team members have the privilege of potentially influencing the decision-making process. This does not necessarily mean that everyone has an equal vote in all team matters (e.g., Covey, 1990; Quick, 1992). This practice naturally fits with the philosophy of early intervention (i.e., supporting parents and service providers as collaborative decision makers).

High Standards and Accountability

The early intervention team is accountable first to families and second to the organizations within which they work and the community at large. Effective teams set standards for quality intervention and develop ways to evaluate their accomplishments. They ask themselves questions such as, "Was there meaningful family involvement in the IFSP process? Did we obtain the resources needed to help a family meet an outcome? Did we develop the brochure to increase awareness of our program?" A team's goal is to meet a family's needs by delivering the best services possible. In responding to the preceding questions, teams must examine their limitations and identify additional knowledge or resources needed to meet their goals. They target areas for change and develop action plans to effect those changes. This continual process of revision and improvement is especially important in a relatively young field such as early intervention.

Appropriate Training, Skills, and Experience of Team Members

Chapter 5 discussed challenges to families in gaining skills to become skillful team members. Professionals often lack training in teaming skills, too. Few preservice programs for the key disciplines in early intervention include content about team dynamics and team building or provide practical experiences in team settings. Few providers have had formal leadership training either, an important team role for many early intervention providers. Most professionals report that they learn the skills on the job. Training in team participation, including skills such as communication, leadership, decision making, and problem solving, is frequently identified as a high-priority early intervention need, and thus is the topic of much in-service training.

Barriers to Effective Teams

As teams strive to acquire the attributes just described, they encounter barriers that reduce their effectiveness. The paragraphs following cite some of the most common barriers.

Scheduling and Time

For early intervention teams, certain barriers occur more frequently than others. For instance, issues related to scheduling and lack of time are often reported as a major barrier to successful teamwork. Finding enough common free time for the team to meet is a challenge for many early intervention teams. This can be especially true if caseloads are high, people work in different agencies, parents work outside of their homes, and some team members travel to homes or work part-time. Yet without this time, many essential activities are sacrificed.

Values Related to Team Participation

Changing values related to team participation present another barrier to successful teamwork. In many sectors of the workplace in the United States, teamwork is becoming the preferred organizational structure. Where once individual initiative and achievement were most highly valued, individual efforts are now viewed within the context of the team (Hicks & Bone, 1990; Quick, 1992; Scholtes, 1988). Individuals who once understood how decisions were made and the boundaries of their work no longer have this clarity. Sources of motivation are changing along with definitions of what constitutes valuable work. In early intervention the context of the team is also changing. Early intervention laws such as the Individuals with Disabilities Education Act (IDEA) of 1990, PL 101–476, suggest that one must act as a member of a team that is family centered, interdisciplinary, and interagency. This is a major change for many practicing early intervention providers. Some may not feel comfortable with these changes and may not want to work within the context of the early intervention team. They may lack commitment to a team process for a variety of reasons such as work-style preferences, lack of team participation skills, bad experiences, or difficulty accepting and adjusting to change.

Differences Among Team Members

Diversity among members of the early intervention team has the potential to both enhance and impede the team's work. Individual team members possess a variety of values, beliefs, knowledge, cultures, education, status, and experience—differences that often complement the diversity of families served by early intervention. Not infrequently, however, these differences can lead to divergent perspectives among team members on how to approach a problem. When conflicts arise, it is important to acknowledge them and work through them. If time is not taken to understand what they mean for the team, frictions can develop and teamwork can suffer.

Inadequate Resources

Inadequate resources for needed services represent another common barrier in early intervention. As mentioned throughout this book, early intervention teams spend a significant proportion of their time helping families identify their needs and instituting plans to accomplish outcomes. It is a tremendous strain on the team when adequate resources such as appropriately trained personnel, funds from health insurance companies, or openings in child care settings are not available. This can be very disturbing to team members who see the needs, know what can be done, and also know that resources are not available. A related barrier in early intervention is obtaining funds. Despite a variety of funding sources that may be appropriate for helping families meet outcomes, discovering what these sources are and how to obtain them can be complicated and time consuming.

Poor Communication Among Members

Poor communication among team members is one of the biggest barriers to effective teamwork. When communication breaks down, nothing gets done or the wrong things get done. In early intervention, this can be disastrous for families: Deadlines for applications are missed, inappropriate treatments are given, or hard feelings develop and relationships deteriorate. Some common communication problems include poor listening, misunderstandings, inability to make decisions, and ignoring team input in decision making. Team activity can also be stalled if people withhold information or hesitate to share new ideas to move the team along.

Poorly Run Meetings

When people attend poorly run meetings, they feel the time they have invested is not well spent. They may not know why they are there, what they are supposed to accomplish, or who will do what when. Consequently, when discussion wanders off course and little or nothing gets done, negative feelings may develop. These problems have particularly striking repercussions for families as team members. Many parents do not feel comfortable in team settings under the best of circumstances. Ambiguous meetings only add to their stress.

The presence of any of these barriers can significantly erode the commitment of team members. As suggested earlier in this discussion, commitment to a common purpose and commitment of time are the overriding prerequisites of all team activities. It is important for team members to understand potential barriers early in the team development process, so that they can respond to them when they occur. Later in this chapter basic skills related to communication, decision making, and conflict management are presented. These skills are tools for avoiding or addressing barriers.

ACTIVITY: *Promoting and Impeding Effective Teamwork*

◆ ◆ ◆   Consider the brief encounter with the Rollins family. Identify the quali-
             ties of effective teams you observed. Also identify the barriers to effective
             teamwork and describe the implications for the Rollins family. ◆

Relationships Among Team Variables

Understanding the relationships among the variables at play within a
team is an important team-building strategy. Team functioning can be
enhanced when individual members understand what they—and other
members—bring to the team, as well as the context in which the team
operates. In early intervention, responses to questions such as, "What
philosophy guides this practice?" "Who is on the team?" "What resources
are available to do the job?" "Who's in charge?" "What do I do?" and
"Where do we do our job?" create the context for the team's work.

One way to decipher the dynamics or interconnections among the
variables contributing to effective teams, and to avoid barriers, is to understand the relationships among the various characteristics of effective
teams. Knowing the intricacies of team dynamics helps members identify
what is going well in the interactions and where interactions are break-
ing down. The section following describes a model commonly used to
show these relationships. The model, depicted in Figure 6.1, is a
schematic of team interactions adopted by Project BRIDGE (Handley &
Spencer, 1986), an educational program designed by the American Academy of Pediatrics for early intervention teams. The model highlights interactions among the characteristics of individual team members, overall
group characteristics, and situational factors. Through unique combinations of these factors, each team emerges with its own "personality"
(Spencer & Coye, 1988).

Individual Characteristics

The first and perhaps most important component of the Project BRIDGE
model comprises individual characteristics. The team begins with the dis-
tinguishing features that each individual brings to the situation—that is,
the individual's special skills, knowledge, experience, personality, and attitudes. Service providers bring training in specific disciplines, as well as
their past personal and professional experiences. Parents bring their personal and professional experiences too, including their expertise about
their child's special needs—often having discussed their child's disability
with more physicians or read more medical journals relevant to their
child's special needs than the service providers on their team. The
Rollinses came to the meeting with questions about a new treatment.
They also came with the experience of having been up with Joey for several days. Some parents have relevant professional training and experi-

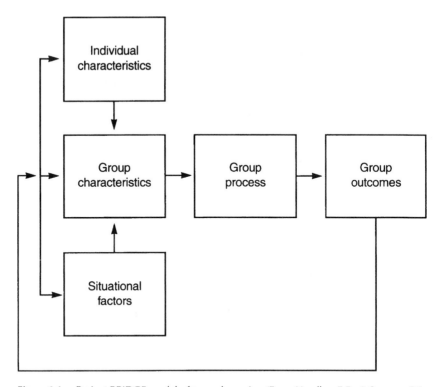

Figure 6.1.   Project BRIDGE model of team dynamics. (From Handley, E.E., & Spencer, P.E. [1986]. *Decision-making for early services: A team approach.* Elk Grove, IL: American Academy of Pediatrics; reprinted by permission.)

ence, just as some other team members have relevant personal experience such as being parents or having a family member with disabilities. All members bring their own unique communication skills, beliefs, values, preferences, needs, and attitudes.

Two important tasks are involved in defining what each individual brings to the team. The first task is for each team member to understand his or her own values, attitudes, experiences, and skills. Some members may be more aware of their values and styles than others and understand how their values and style influence the team process. Many who write about diversity on teams (e.g., Harry, 1992; Locke, 1992; Simons, 1989) contend that the key to understanding what others bring to the team is for each individual to be aware of what he or she brings to the team. Team members must ask themselves, "What are my values and attitudes and how do they merge with the mission and goals of the team?" Self-examination and development of a *personal* mission statement (e.g., Covey, 1990) can aid this process. The purpose of the personal mission statement—which, for example, could be a poem, a list, a story, or a paragraph—is to capture one's unique philosophy or aspirations, one's beliefs and style.

The second important aspect in defining a team's characteristics is to understand what other members bring to the situation. Often our responses to the individuality and differences of other team members are revealed in what we say to ourselves. Menninger and Dugan (1988) have referred to the "silent mind" that works below our level of awareness, resulting in automatic or habitual responses to situations. During the Rollinses' team meeting, several members conveyed negative feelings toward Jacqui and Stuart. It appeared that their own anxieties and stresses took precedence over their concerns for the Rollinses. The key is to be aware of the "silent mind," and to be open to learning new ways to hear and see the characteristics of others.

The IFSP process itself can help team members learn about their own and each other's individual characteristics. For example, members can get acquainted through informal conversations alone, or they can use more formalized checklists. Many teams have had fun using learning- or work-style inventories such as those developed by Meyers-Briggs and Briggs (1980) or Kolb (1985) to discover aspects about themselves and each other. Some of the inventories are standardized and require detailed scoring and interpretation, whereas others require less time and analysis. Most inventories ask participants to circle or rank order adjectives that they feel best describe them at a given point in time. These adjectives tend to fall into one of four categories such as director, doer, thinker, or supporter. The inventories usually have descriptors for the various categories. Many people find they are combinations of more than one category.

ACTIVITY: *Work-Style Inventory*

◆ ◆ ◆   Have members of your team complete a work-style inventory. This can be accomplished independently by obtaining copies of instruments for your team or by inviting a trainer who is familiar with such inventories to meet with your team. Have each team member complete the inventory to determine a predominant work style. Then have each person share the results of his or her inventory with the team. Discuss if the outcomes "fit," and share ideas about what was learned that may benefit the team. Some teams post their results as a reminder of the activity. Remember, most instruments give a point-in-time estimation, and results may vary if taken again.   ◆

Group Characteristics

When people form a team, the collective skills, experiences, and attitudes of the individuals merge into a group personality. The sum of the whole becomes greater than the individual parts. An Ethiopian proverb tells us, "When spider webs unite, they can tie up a lion." As members come together over time, they take on varying roles to accomplish the work of the group. Thus, the group personality changes in response to a variety of circumstances such as how long the team has been together; team size; changes in membership; compatibility or cohesiveness of members; the perceived status of members; and norms that develop within the team. One way to examine these variables is within the context of stages of team development. These stages, as well as the roles of team members, are described in more detail later in this chapter.

Situational Factors

Situational factors consider organizational structure, stability, and goals, as well as sources of support and resources. These define the context for practice. Part H of IDEA has had a dramatic impact on the context of early intervention teams, challenging organizations to examine the philosophies and practices guiding staff's activities. One task that the organizational literature promotes as a framework for team activities is that of developing a mission statement (e.g., Covey, 1990; Quick, 1992). A mission statement should describe the philosophy and primary outcomes that will guide the team's work, based on input from team members. Creating a mission statement is a crucial endeavor in the early stages of team development, giving members a clear understanding of the purposes for a team's activities, as well as guidelines for determining activities that fall within the team's mission.

Another situational factor is that of available resources. Whereas new resources are available for early intervention services, it is generally recognized that needs may be greater than resources. The amount of resources available—that is, human and financial—for team activities has a tremendous impact on team dynamics. Lack of resources can cause significant friction among team members. A clear understanding of resources available and of the priorities for expending them helps a team understand what they have to work with and furthers their ability to make decisions about team activities. Guidelines also help teams identify unmet needs and document activities for future team development. A mission statement could include information about funding priorities. In early intervention it is particularly helpful to build flexibility and creativity into mission statements.

Group Process and Outcomes

Group process is the final component of the Project BRIDGE model. Through the processes of communication, decision making, leadership, and conflict management, a team's individual and group characteristics are interrelated with the situational factors defining the team. These group processes are the driving forces that move the team and give life to it. At every juncture, decisions must be made that either bring the team closer to their outcomes or lead them in another direction. All four processes are basic skills that can be learned and practiced. The final sections of this chapter examine basic skills within each of these driving forces.

Team Development

The literature on team development suggests that teams follow a specific, developmental sequence, with each team moving through the sequence in its own unique way. A framework based on Tuckman's (1965) model of small-group development is frequently used to describe these sequential stages, which are typically called *forming, storming, norming, performing,* and *adjourning* or *reforming.* At each stage, teams must deal with certain issues before they can move on to the next stage. However, teams do not necessarily move through the stages in a linear fashion, because teams are constantly accommodating to changes. Changes in personnel (e.g., losing or adding), the political context (e.g., an election), program funding, governing rules, or family needs can influence a team's developmental process.

Stages of Team Development

The stages of team development and their applications to early intervention are described in the subsections following (e.g., Briggs, 1991; Orelove & Sobsey, 1991; Quick, 1992; SkillPath, 1991).

Forming   The major focus of the *forming* stage is that of "getting acquainted." At this stage, team members meet each other, find out their commonalities, and explore each other's concerns and priorities. They also receive an orientation to the team's purposes and to its mission and goals. They learn how much of the team's purpose and direction is already set and how much team members will have a chance to influence these decisions. Newly forming teams initially tend to rely on direction from a leader or facilitator. For such teams, it is important for all team members, especially parents, to understand that their preferences and style can influence the team's norms. At this stage the size of the group and who is on the team are defined.

Forming teams are often concerned with logistical tasks such as ground rules (e.g., time and place for meetings, attendance, rotation of routine chores) and determination of individual responsibilities. The new group's identity is beginning to form. One task that brings members of a forming team together is that of developing a team name and discussing how it fits with the mission and goals. Discomfort for team members centers around the uncertainties that lie ahead. Clear information and comfortable interactions among members are crucial to this stage. Key questions for team members are the following:

- Who are we?
- Why are we here?
- How should we behave?
- What part will I play?

Storming   The *storming* stage is marked by definition of tasks and roles. This can be a time of instability and conflict. As the team's personality evolves and tasks are undertaken, new issues surface. Members are willing to take risks to share their ideas and assert their priorities. Accompanying these risks are increased possibilities for disagreements. Factions can develop along with struggles for power and control. The overall goals of the team may be challenged, at the same time that deadlines for accomplishing tasks approach.

Status, another dynamic characteristic of the group, may come into play at this point. Status is based on team members' perceptions, which can be influenced by variables such as position, education, values, achievements, salary, employing agency, gender, and behaviors. As mentioned earlier, team members often report differences in status relationships as a barrier to effective team functioning. Status relationships can have both positive and negative effects on interactions among team members. For example, a "high-status" person can establish positive standards for the group or can assume or be granted power in a way that interferes with the team's functioning. A "low-status" person may have difficulty exercising leadership. Teams based on traditional models have often routinely viewed parents as having low status, but on a family-centered team, parents are valued members. Early intervention providers are responsible for ascribing families valued status, and supporting them in gaining the skills required to communicate and express themselves. Members of early intervention teams must also cross traditional barriers to reduce the influence of status relationships on team functioning. Health care providers, educators, social services personnel, and parents have equal value on the early intervention team.

Problem solving and conflict management are critical at the storming stage. The team leader/facilitator plays a key role in guiding the group, to make decisions and resolve differences. Key questions at this stage are the following:

- Do we still think this is a good idea?
- What's going on among us?
- What are we trying to accomplish?
- Why should we change?
- How will we resolve differences?

Norming   During the *norming* stage, the team consolidates into a cohesive, productive group. This period is marked by productivity, positive communication, and feedback. As the team develops, behavioral standards to cover most aspects of a team's functioning emerge. These may include spoken and unspoken norms about punctuality, roles, who talks with whom to accomplish certain functions, what kinds of records are kept, how decisions are made, and so on. These standards provide predictability and comfortable routines for members. People like to know basics—for example, whether they can count on coffee at a morning meeting or should bring their own, as well as norms for more complex tasks such as who will facilitate the meeting. The norming stage can be a very enjoyable time for team members.

Under some circumstances, group norms can impede effective team functioning. For example, some members may always dominate the discussion and skew the group's decisions. A major task of the leader/ facilitator of a norming team is guidance and support, unless the norms become counterproductive. This is a good time for teams to engage in consensus decision making to accomplish team tasks. The key questions are the following:

- How can we work more effectively together?
- How can we support each other?
- What do we understand about our members?
- How can we make good decisions together?

Performing   The *performing* stage focuses on performance, problem solving, and decision making. Interpersonal relationships are stable, and team tasks are clear. Team members are interdependent and have a good sense of whom to count on for what. The team is highly productive, performing quality work. Some members are beginning to look to the future for new challenges. They are interested in identifying new tasks and thinking about creative approaches to accomplish them. If this fails to happen, teams can fall into a rut. Members look to their leader to facilitate activities and to suggest new ideas and resources. The key questions are the following:

- What do we do really well?
- What can we work on?
- What do we want to accomplish?
- What are we thinking about for the future?

Adjourning or Reforming   The last stage is *adjourning* or *reforming*. In this stage team members are either bringing closure to their group's task or choosing new directions. Here the team is reflecting and evaluating. It is a good time to revisit unmet needs of families and unleash the dreams of team members. This can be a feeling-laden process. People may be sad about ending their work together as well as joyful about their accomplishments. Sometimes in the review process old issues and conflicts reemerge. The leader/facilitator of a team in this stage is called upon to recognize the team's accomplishments and give guidance for the future. It is essential that the leader allow feelings to be part of the process. The key questions are the following:

*   What have we accomplished to celebrate?
*   What comes next—closure or new activities?
*   If new activities, what do we want to do?
*   What do we want to change?

ACTIVITY: *Stages of Team Development*

◆ ◆ ◆   Think about the Rollins family.

1. What was your sense about their team's development?
2. Could you identify any norms for that group? Do you think the Rollins family participated in establishing them and understood what they were?
3. What do you think would happen if a newly hired person were present at the meeting?

Now think about a team you have been on.

1. In what stage of development was your team?
2. Were there times when your team was stalled or backed up in the developmental sequence because of changes within or outside of the team? What was that like?
3. What were some of the norms that were established? Did people tend to sit in the same places? Did the same people always talk first? Last? ◆

Implications for Families

Often in early intervention, a new team forms for each family. The family's preferences and the child's needs should determine who is on the team and the size of the team. For some families, the team may consist of three or four people, including the parent, whereas for families of children with complex medical and developmental needs, the team size could be very large if all service providers are included. Families in these circumstances might decide they want to be an integral part of the whole team or only relate to a small portion of key people on the larger team. The Hallmans (see Chapter 5) were interested in being involved with everyone on their team. Each approach has advantages and disadvantages for the family and service providers, and the trade-offs should be considered on an individual family basis. Large teams can easily develop communication and scheduling problems. Although small teams may be more intimate, they may also lack some specific expertise. Preferably, parents should have input into decisions about team size.

Some families have the impression that they joined already-established teams. In these instances, family members may or may not understand the stage of team development they are entering. Team service providers are challenged to communicate to families how the team works together and to establish new communication modes as circumstances warrant.

Another challenge to the development of early intervention teams is that of stability. For a variety of reasons in the rapidly growing and changing area of early intervention, staff turnover can occur frequently. Changes in membership affect group stability, presenting challenges for everyone on the team, especially families who may be receiving less than desirable services. Teams with changing membership may or may not meet often enough or long enough to develop an identity and effective ways of working together. New members are consumed with finding their places on the team, whereas existing members are trying to figure out how to accommodate the changes. Frequent changes tend to keep teams in the early stages of development, never having the opportunity to fully develop their problem-solving skills or to benefit from time to reflect and choose new directions. Conversely, many established early intervention teams have had to reexamine their practices in response to the changing context of early intervention (e.g., Part H of IDEA). These teams, which once may have been stable, enter into an unstable period. From a family's perspective, team stability is essential and a worthy goal for early intervention.

Roles of Team Members

As individuals unite to form a team, they find themselves playing distinct roles. Personality as much as skills, knowledge, discipline, or position influences the team members' roles. Role analysis suggests that individuals play different roles at various times. They may find themselves introducing new ideas at one meeting and drawing conclusions from a series of ideas at another meeting. Individuals may also play more than one role in the same meeting. A team facilitator may find him- or herself supporting others' ideas and encouraging communication among members, as well as setting boundaries to resolve differences.

Multiple sources within the literature have reported similar classifications of team roles (e.g., Landerholm, 1990; Miller, 1991; Quick, 1992; Spencer & Coye, 1988). There is general agreement that some team roles are goal oriented, focusing on task accomplishment, whereas others focus on maintaining the team and on team-building activities. There are also roles that block or hinder team activity. Miller (1991) has referred to the latter as self-oriented roles that meet personal needs. The subsections following discuss these role classifications.

Table 6.1. Task roles of team members

Initiator	Brings a problem to the attention of the team
Information gatherer	Gathers facts relating to a problem
Opinion seeker	Makes sure that all members state their opinions regarding the problem and possible solutions
Clarifier	Makes sure the proposed solution is clear to everyone
Elaborator	Makes sure the proposed solution is examined for all consequences
Energizer	Prods the team into action
Summarizer	Reviews all points related to the ideas
Consensus tester	Asks if the team is ready to decide

Adapted from Handley & Spencer (1986), Landerholm (1990), and Miller (1991).

Task Roles

People in task roles initiate conversation, bring up new ideas, gather information related to the topic, seek opinions from team members, or ask to have information clarified and elaborated so that they and other team members understand the issues. Task-oriented role players may synthesize or organize information to bring a workable idea to the team. There are also task roles that test out whether the team is ready to make a decision, or energize the team into action. Table 6.1 is a summary of task roles adapted from descriptions by Handley and Spencer (1986), Landerholm (1990), and Miller (1991).

Team Maintenance Roles

Team maintenance roles emerge as teams mature or stabilize. Team members' actions build relationships among members to strengthen team activity. Encouragement and participation are key characteristics of maintenance roles. Table 6.2 is a summary of maintenance roles adapted from descriptions by Handley and Spencer (1986), Landerholm (1990), and Miller (1991).

Table 6.2. Maintenance roles of team members

Encourager	Praises and accepts contributions of others
Harmonizer	Relieves conflicts between two members
Compromiser	Backs down in a conflict and compromises
Gatekeeper	Makes sure less assertive members have a chance to express their views
Observer	Offers feedback on team performance in a manner the team can act on
Standard setter	Moves the team to set standards to guide activities
Tension reliever	Uses humor or calls for a break to move away from negative interactions

Adapted from Handley & Spencer (1986), Landerholm (1990), and Miller (1991).

Table 6.3.   Self-oriented roles of team members

Aggressor	Criticizes, attacks, or disagrees aggressively with group, person, or problem
Dominator	Tries to take over and control the group with personal agendas
Withdrawer	Does not participate, may hold side conversations
Blocker	Opposes the group or refuses to move on
Recognition seeker	Talks excessively about personal experiences
Topic jumper	Changes subjects
Self-confessor	Manipulates time with personal feelings and thoughts
Devil's advocate	Constantly takes opposing view
Jokester	Uses irreverent jokes or cynical humor

Adapted from Handley & Spencer (1986) and Miller (1991).

Roles to Meet Personal Needs

Roles to meet personal needs often block team progress. Team members assume self-oriented roles for a variety of reasons, sometimes as the result of a major difference of opinion about the overall goal of the group or owing to a member's deeply held values and beliefs. People may also block progress because of discomfort on the team, personality conflicts, or unmet needs in other areas of their lives. Members may tend to play these roles on all teams, or only as a result of very specific circumstances on a particular team. Table 6.3 is a summary of self-oriented roles adapted from descriptions by Handley and Spencer (1986) and Miller (1991).

ACTIVITY: *Rollins Meeting Follow-Up Skit*

◆ ◆ ◆   A return visit with the team from the Seneca Early Intervention Program (minus the Rollinses) illustrates many of the dynamics at play within one aspect of the early intervention process, the IFSP review. The outcome of the Rollinses' Wednesday morning meeting was that they wanted more physical therapy. The following skit[1] brings to life a meeting in which the team struggles with this request. Read or act out the skit to examine a variety of issues that face the Rollinses' team.

The Rollins Family Wants More Physical Therapy

Setting: Monthly staff meeting at the Seneca Early Intervention Program.
Issue: The Rollinses have requested physical therapy three times a week to implement a new treatment. Staff perceive that resources do not currently permit the requested intensity of service.
Purpose of the meeting: To discuss the Rollinses' request as a staff, without parents present.

---

[1]Written and performed by Peggy Rosin, George S. Jesien, Linda I. Tuchman, and Amy D. Whitehead, of the Wisconsin Family-Centered Inservice Project, Waisman Center University Affiliated Program, Madison, Wisconsin, June 1992.

Staff present:

Amy Primary Colors, the early childhood teacher

Barb Oldtimer, the social worker/service coordinator

George Handstand, the physical therapist

Linda C. Oordinator, the program coordinator and speech-language pathologist

Barb: I was afraid this would happen. The outcome of Wednesday's meeting was that the Rollinses want more physical therapy. I think it's because of something they read or maybe they didn't like the results of the recent assessment we did. Now they want to up their physical therapy from once a week to three times a week.

George: (*Shaking his head*) There's no way, there's just no way, I can't do it! I only work half time and my schedule's completely filled. I do most of my paperwork at home on my own time as it is.

Amy: You do work very hard and I know kids benefit from your work.

Barb: Kids benefit from all of our work. We've all always had heavy caseloads and done our paperwork at home. I remember when I was in juvenile justice and I had hundreds of cases of families in crises.

George: (*A little disgusted*) Oh, Barb, not the families in crises stories again!

Linda: I know it's not going to be easy, but we do need to find a way of dealing with this request. We may be getting more requests like this in the future.

Barb: I bet not only the Rollinses, but the Andersons, Rosemans, Johnsons, and Blackhawks will be asking tomorrow. Just wait. Today they're asking for physical therapy, tomorrow nursing. And plus look at our salaries! Linda, did you talk to the county administrator about our salary schedules?

Linda: I've been meaning to tell you, I don't have any news on the salary schedule. I think they're stalling because they don't know what to do with our requests. I'll be meeting with. . . .

Amy: We can talk about the salaries at the meeting next week. What are we going to do about this problem? I'm concerned we're not going to figure this out before our meeting is over.

Barb: I'm not sure we'll ever figure this out.

Linda: Perhaps going to the home three times a week isn't the only way to respond to the Rollinses' request.

Barb: In the old days we used to schedule intensive blocks of time rather than once-a-week slots. We found it more efficient for helping some children.

Amy: (*To George*) Don't you drive by the house on your way to work every day? Couldn't you fit in a couple more stops each week?

Barb: Yes, if you're really dedicated you would. We used to get up at 5 A.M., just to get there in the morning.

George: (*Pulls out a chart with colored dots*) Now here I've got 20 children with 15 minutes for setup and 5 minutes to talk to parents. As far as I can see, the most I've got is two half-hour slots open.

Linda: I don't think we should jump to this conclusion without looking at more options.

Amy: Why don't we invite the Rollinses to come and talk to us about what they were thinking and different ways we could meet their needs.

All: (*Look quizzically as if an idea for a solution may be emerging.*)

1. What is your reaction to the skit?
2. How did the individual characteristics of each team member add to or block the team's functioning?
3. Can you describe the roles the members played on the team?
4. How did Barb Oldtimer impede the team's decision-making process?
5. How did the issue of resources (time and money) affect the team's discussion?
6. Did anyone take the leadership role? How might Linda have kept Barb from derailing the focus of the meeting? ◆

COMMUNICATION SKILLS TO ENHANCE TEAM BUILDING

"I know you believe you understand what you think I said,
but I'm not sure you realize that what you heard is not what I meant."

—Anonymous

Overhearing a conversation between two people, one might be struck by the incredible complexity of their communication. How do these conversational partners know what to say next? What to add to the topic? When to change the topic? How much explanation or detail to give? Communication in groups is even more complex.

To communicate, a person sends an encoded message. Before speaking, the person passes the message through his or her perceptual filters, formed by past experience, thoughts, and values. The listener responds not only to the speaker's words but also to voice and body language. In interpreting the message, the listener passes it through his or her own perceptual filters. It is easy to see how the message can be misconstrued. This is especially true with telephone communication because nonverbal cues are not available. For communication to be effective, each person must fully understand the message intended by the other.

Effective communication is a learned skill. It takes practice. To become a better communicator, it is helpful to be aware of the various components of the communication process: What keeps it going? Where does it fall apart? Simons (1989) described four basic communication acts that frequently occur within team interactions.

Team members ask others to do things and get asked to do things. This could include tasks such as attending a meeting, participating in an evaluation, making a telephone call, or outlining decisions to be made.

Team members promise each other things they will or will not do. For example, team members may agree to take notes, make a telephone call, get the physician's referral, make a home visit, or write a letter.

Team members tell each other what they believe to be true or false. Team members may share belief statements such as, "Early intervention is effective," "Families know their children well," "All eligible children should receive early intervention services," or "Teamwork takes too much time and effort."

Team members commit themselves to a set of attitudes, directions, definitions, or situational factors. This may include commitment to practices such as making early intervention family centered, giving families choices over services, or the team's use of a transdisciplinary approach.

When people understand these basic communication acts, a team functions well. When misunderstandings occur, team functioning breaks down. One of the major benefits of good communication is that it prevents or at least minimizes the effects of conflict. The remainder of this section focuses on practical applications of basic communication skills to enhance team functioning.

Communication Process Model

The Communication Process Model, developed at the University of Wisconsin–Madison (Dean of Students Office, 1991), is one means to teach people how to communicate more effectively. The model is based on several assumptions about how people communicate, as follows:

Communication is a circular rather than a linear process. Each message is a response to a situation (internal or external) or to cues from the other person.

The degree to which an individual is self-aware affects the degree to which that person can present him- or herself. An important foundation of interpersonal communication is to nurture individual well-being.

The result of each interpersonal interaction is the product of both persons involved. An individual can take responsibility only for his or her own contribution to the communicative interaction.

Effective communication involves risks.

Communication is central to everything we do.

The Communication Process Model (Dean of Students Office, 1991) includes six components: self-awareness, listening, responding, assertiveness, checking for understanding, and conflict management (see Figure 6.2). A

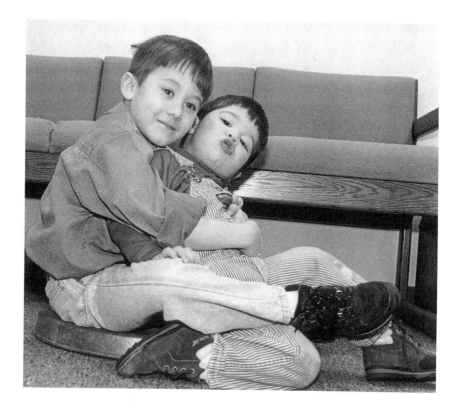

description of the first five components of the model follows. The model's final component, managing conflict, is discussed at the end of this section.

Self-Awareness

The first component, and the model's foundation, is self-awareness. Self-awareness is an important prerequisite to understanding and effecting interactions with others. Covey (1990) has written that individuals must know and understand themselves to like themselves and to present themselves confidently to others. A self-aware person has more to offer others in the interdependent setting of a team. Brahms (1995) wrote, "When I am aware of the attitudes, values, opinions or the agenda of the person with whom I am in dialogue, I frequently am less cautious and protective of my own opinions and ideas" (p. 6A). "Self-skills" include awareness of one's own communication patterns, past experiences, values, beliefs, needs, goals, ability to empathize, and listening and responding skills. During this phase of the model, individuals learn to realize that each person can be responsible only for his or her part of a communica-

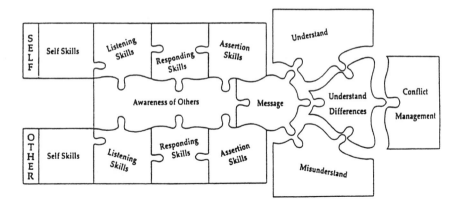

Figure 6.2. Communication Process Model. (From Dean of Students Office. [1991]. *Communication skills trainer's manual.* Madison: University of Wisconsin–Madison, Dean of Students Office; reprinted by permission.)

tive exchange. Because early intervention is a set of values-based services, self-awareness is extremely important. Members of early intervention teams need to be able to answer the following question for themselves: "Would I be willing to answer the questions that I'm asking of another team member—family or professional?"

Listening

The second component of the Communication Process Model is that of listening. Covey (1990) has advocated seeking understanding before seeking to be understood. Effective listening is the basis for understanding another's messages (see Table 6.4 for a list of characteristics of good

Table 6.4. Characteristics of good listening

1. Give the other an opportunity to talk.
2. Establish an environment where the other person feels comfortable speaking.
3. Demonstrate interest by asking appropriate questions.
4. Lead the other to talk.
5. Show interest through your body language.
6. Attend to the content, not just the delivery of the message.
7. Listen to the complete message.
8. Deal effectively with emotionally charged language.
9. Listen for the main idea.
10. Deal effectively with others' listening roadblocks.
11. Identify areas of common experience and agreement.
12. Practice listening.

From Herman, P. (assisted by Murphy, M.). (1990). *Parent involvement resource manual: Comprehensive materials for teaching parent involvement.* Madison: Wisconsin Council on Developmental Disabilities; reprinted by permission.

listening). Listening is far more complex than it first appears. Skills such as being attentive, being impartial, and listening for feelings (Edelman, Greenland, & Mills, 1992) require practice. Attention must be paid to both the verbal and nonverbal messages being sent by the speaker. Good listeners also must learn to avoid common roadblocks that inhibit effective listening. Some of these are listed in Table 6.5.

Responding

Responding is the third component of the Communication Process Model. The listener's response demonstrates whether he or she has in fact listened to the speaker. The listener reflects both the content, or meaning, and the feeling of the message. When the message has strong emotional content, it is important to acknowledge that emotion and to attempt to reconcile any differences between what is said and how it is said. Responding skills help ensure that the original message has been understood. Here the listener reflects feelings and meanings (e.g., "I heard you say—you are upset about. . .or. . .want to. . . ."); he or she paraphrases (e.g., "It sounds like you have concerns about. . . ."); he or she questions (e.g., "Do you think. . . ?"); he or she clarifies (e.g., "Could you tell me more about. . . ?"); and he or she summarizes or interprets the message to ensure that he or she understands the sender's message (e.g., "This is what I believe you are saying. . . ."). Turn taking and watching for cues to continue listening or to respond are integral parts of responding.

ACTIVITY: *Listening and Responding Skills*

◆◆◆   The following encounter with Jacqui Rollins and Barbara Lander provides an opportunity to practice five skills associated with reflective listening and responding. These skills are reflecting feelings and meanings, paraphrasing, questioning, clarifying, and summarizing or interpreting for understanding. Find a partner to play out the roles begun in the script following. One partner will take on Jacqui's role and the other will be Barbara. Begin by reading the script. Continue the conversation through role play. Attempt to use the skills of reflective listening and responding described earlier. Hint: Barbara has the feeling that Jacqui is upset.

Excerpted Conversation

In the IFSP review of Joey's progress, the speech-language pathologist, Linda, described Joey's eating skills. Barb and Jacqui are discussing Linda's findings in the skit below.

Jacqui: So Joey's not drinking from a cup yet, and most kids are by his age. Is that right?

Barb: Yes, but Joey may need to work on some other skills before he'll be ready to drink from a cup.

Table 6.5.   Roadblocks to listening

1. *Comparing* what the speaker says to him- or herself or to others.
2. *Rehearsing* what you will say in response to the speaker.
3. *Mind reading* what the speaker is *really* feeling or thinking.
4. *Judging* the merits of what the speaker says or how it is said.
5. *Identifying* what the speaker says with personal experience.
6. *Advising* the speaker and providing solutions without being asked.
7. *Diverting* the speaker by changing the subject, distracting him or her from the topic.
8. *Being right* in one's position or idea, leaving no room for listening to the other's perspective.
9. *Placating* the speaker by agreeing with him or her without being involved in what is said.

Adapted from Wolfe, Petty, & McNellis (1990).

Jacqui: So he's not ready to do it, but he should be doing it for his age. It's another way that he's delayed, in addition to not walking. I see.

(*Jacqui's voice and body both suggest that she is feeling sad. She has slumped in her chair, and her voice has gotten much softer with a slight quiver.*)

I really need to take a break now, if that's okay?
Barb: Sure. Let's take a 10-minute break.

Consider the following questions:

1. How did it feel to be a reflective listener and responder, or to be listened to and responded to in that way?
2. Consider other real-life situations. Think of times when you felt heard, and used good responding skills.
3. Discuss roadblocks and effective strategies for using these skills.   ◆

Assertiveness

The model's fourth component is assertiveness. Assertiveness means "delivering a message in a positive and confident manner, with the knowledge that we are personally responsible for our statements and actions" (Dean of Students Office, 1991, p. 81). Assertiveness helps clarify communication blocks and misunderstandings. When a situation calls for assertiveness, the model suggests a three-part assertion message:

Behavior:	When you....
+	
Feelings:	I feel....
+	
Effects:	because....

Some points to consider when making assertions include being direct and to the point, and clearly stating the perceived problem. Also choose words and maintain a tone of voice and body language that convey an interest in working things out, not placing blame. Then be sure to give the other person a chance to respond.

An assertion is an opportunity to get a message across. There are no guarantees about how an assertion will be received. Covey (1990) writes that how well assertions are received depends on what type of goodwill has been built up between the parties. Goodwill can be built among team members when they help each other out—"I'll listen to you. . .I'll fill out this form. . .I'll find out what we can do. . . ." When there is goodwill among team members, the person asserting him- or herself is more likely to get the response he or she wants. If the relationship is strained, there is less flexibility. The Rollinses' lateness may or may not be an issue for the team. A team member may say to the Rollinses, "When you are late to meetings, I start to feel anxious because I fear it will throw my schedule off for the whole day." The Rollinses may or may not be able to comfortably respond to this.

Checking for Understanding

The fifth component of the Communication Process Model is checking out whether the message has been understood. If the message has not been comprehended, then the communicators need to return to earlier phases of the model to discover why the breakdown occurred. If the message has been understood, and there is agreement on the issue, then communication has been successful. If the message has been understood, but there is disagreement on the issue, then there is conflict to be managed.

In the listening and responding processes, it is helpful to send effective messages to ensure understanding (e.g., Bolton, 1979; Edelman et al., 1992). Effective messages are complete and specific, and the verbal and the nonverbal components are congruent. It is okay to be redundant, sending the same message more than once, and asking for feedback to find out if the message was received. When talking about feelings, own them, and give them a name, action, or figure of speech. When describing others' behaviors, avoid evaluating or interpreting them.

Decision-Making Process and Leadership

Decision making is a structured communication process, building on many communication skills already discussed in this chapter. Adopting a systematic process for making decisions can improve team effectiveness. The Rollins team would clearly benefit from a more systematic way to respond to Stuart's and Jacqui's concerns. A variety of decision-making models are applicable to early intervention teams (e.g., Briggs, 1991; Handley & Spencer, 1986; Miller, 1991). Most have similar stages such as identifying the problem, generating alternatives, and developing, implementing, and evaluating a plan. It is the organizational structure and leadership style that distinguish specific aspects of the process, such as who decides which alternatives will be chosen. The five-step process of decision making outlined next is based on the Project BRIDGE (Handley & Spencer, 1986) model.

Identifying the Problem

Problem identification is crucial to the outcome of the process. Unless the problem is clearly stated, the response may address the wrong issue. Issues should be framed in a positive way, or with a specified outcome. For example, "We want to increase our planning time" is preferable to "We never have enough planning time." In the Rollinses' situation, the issue may be, "What options are available to support the Rollins family's request for more physical therapy?" This keeps the team's energies positively focused. During this phase, information is gathered through team discussion, needs assessments, questionnaires, and other methods. The team examines the data and defines the issue to be addressed. Success is more likely if the team chooses an issue that is possible and within members' control. If some stakeholders are not present, the team may postpone actions until they are available. It is helpful to bring absent members up to date for future meetings.

Generating Alternatives

After the problem is clearly defined, the team generates possible strategies to address the problem. All team members, especially parents, should be encouraged to offer suggestions. Brainstorming is often used at this stage to provide a number of creative ideas in a short amount of time. There are numerous ways to conduct brainstorming; some are parallel, and some are interactive (Zemke, 1993). Both types can vary the level of anonymity and sequence in the process. For example, in interactive brainstorming, participants can write their responses and share them back and forth with each other, or they can verbally share ideas. In a parallel structure, participants complete their input simultaneously. All media (e.g., drawing, writing, talking) are possible. A few rules apply: No criticism, evaluation, or judgment is allowed during brainstorming; building on or combining ideas is fine; and the atmosphere must be one of trust and acceptance so that all team members feel comfortable generating as many associated ideas as possible. Participants are encouraged to drop their own sensors in order to release their most creative ideas. Research shows that quantity is more important than quality (Zemke, 1993). This means that the more ideas on the table, no matter how offbeat, the more likely a group is to come up with creative, workable ideas. Imagine all the possibilities for helping the Rollinses decide how the new treatment might fit into their and Joey's routines.

Selecting Alternatives

During the selecting alternatives step, each alternative is discussed, judged, and evaluated, and one or more or a combination of ideas is selected. Evaluation of alternatives might be based on criteria such as feasibility, legal and ethical considerations, anticipated effectiveness, and consequences beyond solving the problem. When tough decisions must be made, it is good to have a system for evaluating alternatives. It is helpful to gather all the important information and discuss the consequences for selecting or not selecting the various alternatives. It may be desirable to pick the alternative with the lowest risk, the best chance for success, or the one that will satisfy the most people. Once all the options have been thoroughly analyzed, it is useful to rank them, either as a group or individually. Eventually, it is important to come to agreement.

Decision-Making Approach

The manner in which agreement is achieved will depend on a team's organizational structure and leadership. When it comes to selecting alternatives and committing resources, decisions can be made in a number of ways. Decisions may be made by consensus; by majority; unilaterally by a team leader; or by a delegation of selected members such as parents in early intervention. The way decisions are made varies with the circumstances. The person with the final decision-making authority may or may not be present at the table. In some instances consensus may rule, and in others a unilateral decision holds. Table 6.6 summarizes four leadership styles along with the key leadership tasks of each, and the implications for team members (Rees, 1991).

The five-step decision-making process may appear different within each of these styles. In early intervention, it is preferable for members to collaborate in decision making. Consensus, by which the team engages in a process to come to a common decision, is often the best way to accomplish this. In consensus not everyone gets his or her way, but all end by agreeing, even if it is agreeing to disagree. The major disadvantage of consensus is that to reach full agreement, the outcome may include compromises that do not fully satisfy anyone.

One model of team organization and decision making that is becoming popular in American society is the self-management model (e.g., Hicks & Bone, 1990; Scholtes, 1988). This model is built around collaborative participation, and in many ways is compatible with philosophies inherent in early intervention. Early intervention team members may benefit from learning more about the model and its applicability to early intervention. A self-managing team functions with varying degrees of autonomy and without a visible manager. Control comes from within the group. Team members assume management and decision-making responsibility in addition to their specific jobs such as speech-language pathologist. These new responsibilities are shared among team members—requiring new learning for some—and may include planning, organizing, directing, and monitoring team tasks and administrative functions (Hicks & Bone, 1990).

Developing the Action Plan

Action plans are developed to record decisions made by the team. Flipcharts, laptop computers, sticky notes, or other recording methods can be helpful in facilitating the development of the written plan. An effective plan

Table 6.6.   Styles of leadership

Leader functions	Group needs met	Leader tasks	Team-member tasks
Lead with a clear purpose.	• Common goals • Attention to content • Leadership	• Set boundaries. • Interpret company goals. • Facilitate team's setting of its own goals. • Evaluate and track progress toward goals.	• Ask questions to test own understanding. • Participate in setting goals for team. • Help leader track and evaluate progress toward goals.
Empower to participate.	• High level of involvement of all members • Maintenance of self-esteem • Leadership • Respect for differences • Trust	• Ask questions. • Listen. • Show understanding. • Summarize. • Seek divergent viewpoints. • Record ideas.	• Contribute ideas from own experience and knowledge. • Listen to others. • Build on others' ideas. • Ask questions. • Think creatively.
Aim for consensus.	• Constructive conflict resolution • Power within group to make decisions • Leadership • Trust	• Use group-process techniques (brainstorming, problem solving, prioritization, etc.). • Ask questions. • Listen. • Seek common interests. • Summarize. • Confront in constructive way.	• Focus on common interests and goals. • Listen to and consider others' ideas. • Make own needs known. • Disagree in constructive way.
Direct the process.	• Attention to process • Leadership • Trust	• Give clear directions. • Intervene to keep group on track. • Read group and adjust. • Remain neutral. • Suggest alternate processes to help group achieve goal.	• Listen. • Keep purpose in mind. • Stay focused on objective. • Use own energy and enthusiasm to help process along.

addresses the five Ws. It includes the problem as stated in the first stage of the decision-making process. It lists strategies to address challenges, and resources available to achieve the desired outcome. If all necessary resources are not available, the plan includes strategies for seeking additional resources. The plan specifies who is responsible for each action to be taken, the time line, and an evaluation and monitoring plan. It is helpful for each team member to leave the planning meeting with a written copy of the action plan (or to receive one shortly after the meeting). This clarifies team members' roles in relation to the outcome and helps to keep people on task.

Implementing the Plan

In the implementation stage, all actions focus on achieving the objectives specified in the plan. Planned contacts are made and necessary resources are sought and put in place. This is a time of action, with ongoing communication among key players. Too often, efforts to execute even the best of plans fall off in the implementation phase. People lose contact with each other or get too busy. If resources are not found, action is further compromised and commitment dwindles. Informal communication networks can be particularly helpful in keeping the plan alive. These networks allow team members to share progress and concerns along the way. If things are going well, people know to proceed as planned. If things are not progressing as intended, the team should evaluate what has occurred and find ways to get back on track.

Monitoring the Plan

Monitoring plays an important role in keeping the team focused on achieving planned activities. Action plans specify times and methods for convening the team to formally evaluate progress. In the IFSP process this could be the 6-month or annual review. However, the team can be reconvened before the specified time if any member thinks the plan is not progressing as intended. This is the value of ongoing, informal communication. Previous steps in the decision-making process should be reviewed to pinpoint the source of the difficulty. For example, new information may lead the team to return to Step 1 and redefine the issue. The decision-making process is best visualized as circular, not linear. Team members may continue working toward an outcome while occasionally returning to earlier steps to clarify issues, reassign responsibility, adjust time lines, and so forth.

ACTIVITY: *Problem-Solving with the Rollins Family*

◆ ◆ ◆   Consider how badly things are going for the Rollinses and the rest of the team. The Wednesday morning meeting was a disaster. The subsequent team meeting to discuss the request for more physical therapy was also confusing. Finally the team is reconvening with the Rollinses to engage in a problem-solving session to come up with a plan to move their team forward.

1. Apply the five-step decision-making process to identify the issues and generate a workable plan of action, including strategies for implementing and monitoring proposed actions.
2. If you have access to a team, role-play this activity with them. You may want to choose roles (e.g., Barbara—the service coordinator, Stuart—Joey's father, Jacqui—Joey's mother, George—the physical therapist) and develop your plan as a role play. Prior to beginning the process decide how decisions will be made—by consensus, majority, team facilitator, or the parents. ◆

Communication Skills for Running Effective Meetings

Members of early intervention teams—those with formal leadership roles as well as others—carry out numerous management roles. Facilitating or conducting meetings is one management task that early intervention service providers are often called upon to perform. The organization of the meeting and communications from the facilitator influence the outcome. Good meetings have five well-organized and well-run components: preplanning, a beginning, a middle, an ending, and follow-up activities. Good preplanning and preparation can make the difference between a successful meeting and a failure. A good meeting facilitator is organized for the meeting and can focus his or her attention on interactions within the meeting (e.g., Quick, 1992; Swan & Morgan, 1993). People know when and where the meeting will be held and why it is being held. Materials are prepared in advance, and the room is arranged so that people can see each other to promote interactions. The facilitator begins the meeting with introductions or some other warm-up activity to create a good atmosphere. During the meeting, the facilitator keeps the group focused on the meeting's purpose(s) and moves through the agenda while also admitting reactions from the group; responds to problems as they occur and ensures that people are heard; shares information and asks questions to create a feedback loop; brings closure to the meeting (e.g., summarizes what has occurred, establishes next steps) and creates a "to do" follow-up list (Swan & Morgan, 1993); and, finally, follows through with activities on the "to do" list, further increasing his or her credibility for future meetings. Table 6.7 details organizational strategies and communication skills for facilitators to consider when planning and running a meeting.

ACTIVITY: *Improving Team Meetings*

◆ ◆ ◆   The staff of the Seneca Early Intervention Program want to work on improving their team's meetings. Members are unclear on their roles and of the resources available to them, they are unsure of agendas, and their meetings lack strong leadership. Barb intends to call the team together to

Table 6.7.   Tips for planning and running a meeting

Preplanning
1.   Plan the meeting carefully.
>   **What?**
>   –do you want to accomplish at this meeting or series of meetings? Why?
>   –roles and responsibilities will individuals have?
>   –materials need to be prepared (e.g., agenda, minutes of prior meetings, reports)?
>   –decision-making process will be used?
>   **Who?**
>   –should be there?
>   –should be represented?
>   –will facilitate the meeting?
>   –will have power and authority to make decisions?
>   –will make presentations?
>   –will take notes?
>   –will prepare materials?
>   –will notify participants?
>   –will reserve meeting space?
>   **When?**
>   –will the meeting be held?
>   –will the agenda go out?
>   –will participants be notified?
>   **Where?**
>   –will the meeting be held?
>   **How?**
>   –will records be kept?
>   –will decisions be made?
2.   Notify participants of the meeting.
3.   Prepare and send out an agenda in advance (if appropriate).
4.   Arrive early to set up the meeting room.

Running the meeting: The beginning
1.   Start on time.
2.   Have participants introduce themselves; consider including a warm-up activity.
3.   Pass out materials.
4.   Review, revise, and order the agenda.
5.   Discuss time limits and set limits if appropriate.
6.   Review activities of previous meeting(s).

Running the meeting: The middle
1.   Focus discussion on agenda item(s).
2.   Move the group toward action and/or decisions.
3.   Allow participants to be heard.
4.   Respond to stresses as they occur.
5.   Monitor the time and take a break, if needed.

(continued)

Table 6.7. (*continued*)

Running the meeting: The end

1. Establish future actions (who, what, when).
2. Review group decisions and actions. Prepare a "to do" list.
3. Set the date and place for the next meeting.
4. End on time, bringing closure to activity.
5. Clean up the room.

Following up

1. Prepare minutes if appropriate.
2. Follow up on "to do" list.
3. Begin to plan for the next meeting.

Adapted from Bruder, Lippman, Bologna, & Derrickson (1991); Mealy (1984); and SkillPath (1991).

directly address some of these issues. Imagine you are at the meeting and want to help the team improve their meetings.

1. Create a checklist with practices that you think will increase the effectiveness of the team's meetings. Be specific; make no assumptions.
2. What will happen during preplanning? At the beginning, middle, and end of the meeting? What will be done as follow-up?
3. If you are working on a team, consider this activity for your own team, using a decision-making framework to agree on the points. ◆

One of the most challenging tasks for a team facilitator is that of responding to conflicts that occur during the meeting. As pointed out in this chapter, conflict is an inevitable part of team meetings. Much of the conflict can be attributed to the various previously described blocking roles (see Miller, 1991). Team facilitators and other team members can use a number of skills to minimize these blocking roles. Swan and Morgan (1993) offer several practical strategies for team facilitators. These are described in the subsections following.

The Monopolizer

To minimize opportunities for a team member to monopolize the meeting, the facilitator can assert some control over the way team members contribute to the meeting. The facilitator can set time limits on each person's comments or have members take turns giving input. The facilitator can stress the importance of relevant comments and gain group consensus or unilaterally decide to cut off comments irrelevant to the topic. He or she can also engage the rest of the team in giving feedback to each other about their participation.

The Withdrawer

When a person withdraws, the facilitator may want to try to get to know that person outside of a team meeting to learn about his or her interests and concerns. There may be simple activities that feel safe and will draw that person into the team's interactions. It may be a matter of self-confidence in asserting ideas or uncertainty about what is acceptable in the group. The withdrawer may also need time to observe to feel more comfortable in participating.

The Aggressor

With aggressive team members, good conflict management skills are necessary. The first rule is to try to stay calm and avoid battles. There may be a specific reason for the aggression. Stuart Rollins is not typically confrontational, but was more so than usual after a bad night. It is important for the facilitator to give the aggressive person a chance to explain and to clarify his or her concerns. More listening than acting may be helpful. Facilitators should not make hasty decisions and should speak only for themselves. They should try to diffuse tensions between individuals and focus attention on the issues.

The Blocker

The oppositional behaviors of the blocker require substantial redirecting by the team facilitator and other team members. A facilitator can use responding skills to acknowledge the comments and reframe them in a more positive light. The facilitator or another team member can put the ownership of irrelevant or interfering issues back on the blocker. The team can move the focus off the blocker and demonstrate positive approaches for responding to difficult issues. Citing of concrete examples to show how closure has been brought to subjects can also be helpful.

More About Conflict Management

"A man convinced against his will is still of the same opinion."

—Author Unknown

Inevitable. . .a natural part of life. . .a catalyst for change. . .exhausting. . .time consuming. . .stressful. These are only a few of the adjectives commonly associated with the word *conflict*. This chapter has pointed out potential sources of conflict as well as strategies for preventing or minimizing conflict. Change, even when exciting, carries potential for conflict. Part H of IDEA has created important changes in the philosophy and practice of early intervention. Along with modifications in professional roles and ways of interacting comes the potential for conflict in many arenas—interpersonal, team, organization, and interagency, to name a few. The challenge is not to avoid conflict because it is an inevitable part of life, but to handle it constructively as an opportunity for growth and progress.

It is essential to identify the source of a conflict in order to resolve it. It is also helpful to identify who is involved by considering the following questions: Do I own this problem or does someone else? If I don't own it, what role can I take to move it along? If I own the problem, what can I do to get what I want? If the conflict is the result of a misunderstanding, the Communication Process Model can be used to clarify communication. If the conflict is based on differences in values, the team may need to acknowledge and accept the differences and "agree to disagree." A conflict resulting from lack of information may be resolved by providing the missing information. The decision-making process may be helpful if the conflict occurs because of differences in perceived need or perspective. When conflict occurs because individuals feel a lack of control over situations, it is helpful to analyze where influence can be asserted (Covey, 1990). The Rollinses may not be able to have physical therapy three times a week, but they may be able to integrate the new treatment into all aspects of Joey's program with consultation from a therapist who specializes in the new treatment. They may end up getting assistance from the program in meeting their desire to try out the new treatment, even if it is not physically possible to add another day of physical therapy.

Managing conflicts is more challenging than making decisions, because people are more emotionally involved in conflict. People respond to conflict in a variety of ways, usually to protect themselves in some fashion or another. Anger and fear lead to a whole host of behaviors, some more constructive than others. Some people pull away from the conflict, avoiding it, smoothing it over, moving out of its way, or letting someone else handle it. Others confront it directly, some more aggressively than others.

Conflict is usually triggered by people's perceptions, which are largely based on their past experiences and values. The same event may seem insignificant to one person but major to another. Some people have little tolerance for any behavior that falls outside of their worldview, whereas others find conflict only in extreme situations. In addition, different types of things may bother the same person under different circumstances. It was unusual for Jacqui to have become so quiet and for Stuart to have acted so aggressively at the initial IFSP review meeting. The stress of the situation was the likely reason, but there may have been other reasons, such as their fear about Joey's developmental progress. Under other circumstances, it might have been lack of trust or poor communication with staff at the center. It is important to consider all of the possible reasons leading to conflict in order to resolve differences.

Kindler (1988) offered four guiding principles for resolving conflicts:

Preserve dignity and self-respect. Focus on the issues rather than on team members' personalities. Identify the merits of various arguments and evaluate according to these, not according to whose position is most popular or who has the most pull. It takes skill to identify the issues, and practice to stay focused on those issues, rather than on personalities.

Listen with empathy. Listen with neutrality, with the goal of understanding the other person's perspective. Attempt to suspend your position as you listen, avoiding roadblocks that can interfere with listening. Try the "shoes" test: How does it feel to be in the other person's shoes? This is also a learned skill. Good listening in nonconflictual situations is good practice for a conflict situation.

Don't expect to change the behaviors of others. An individual can be responsible only for his or her own behavior. An individual can watch and monitor his or her own behavior in an effort to influence the outcome of a conflictual situation. Whereas the individual cannot change others, he or she can assert influence within the interdependent team process. It is useful to be aware of what might trigger a reaction that may lead to conflict, and then concentrate on one's own performance. Notice what behaviors exacerbate the conflict and which ones work toward reconciliation.

Express independent perspectives. It is imperative that each team member have the opportunity for his or her perspective to be heard and understood by the team. Individuals must share what they want, even if it flies in the face of popular opinion. If this is difficult, team members are advised to seek support outside the situation in order to find the courage to act on their convictions. Even if a team member is prepared to accept an alternative or compromising position, it is important to ensure that members understand a particular point of view. Individuals should not give way completely to positions that betray their belief systems. In evaluating various positions, picture what could happen with each alternative. What are the consequences, positive and negative, of each position? Know what is and is not acceptable.

The goal of conflict is to achieve a win–win situation (e.g., Bolton, 1979; Covey, 1990; Kinder, 1988), that is, for all key stakeholders to find something satisfactory in the solution. This is most likely to occur when communication is effective and trust levels are high. Often, conflict management involves compromises. Sometimes conflict is not resolved, especially if it arises out of strong beliefs that are not popularly held by the majority of people with whom one comes into contact. At times, it is important to hold onto those beliefs. It should be easy to understand why families in early intervention who are advocating for their children feel so strongly about what they want. Often systems barriers and accompanying miscommunications lead to much of the conflict. For professionals in early intervention, conflicts may emerge over disciplinary or agency boundaries. Most of these difficulties result from lack of experience in "doing things differently." It is helpful to believe that most people enter into early intervention with good intentions. Frequently, it is the forces that people feel powerless to influence that are the source of much conflict. The challenge is to find points of influence and then apply the communication skills offered throughout this chapter.

SUMMARY

This chapter examines the numerous, intricately woven components that define a team—the nerve center that stimulates and maintains the heart, and troubleshoots when problems arise. The Rollins family and other members of the Seneca Early Intervention Program team illustrated many of these dynamics. The examples from the Rollins family study tended to demonstrate what not to do, thus providing opportunities for readers to practice the positive skills of team dynamics discussed in the chapter. Practical ideas for enhancing communication and for building more effective early intervention teams were offered throughout; skills that promote positive interactions were introduced; and strategies for responding to behaviors that impede teamwork were suggested. The challenge is to remain both self-aware and aware of interactions within the team. This takes time, commitment, and practice; most of the techniques discussed in this chapter are learned. A willingness to listen and to allow others to be heard, as well as ongoing efforts at understanding, formed the foundation for most skills. These universal communication skills are continually cited by parents as characteristics that make them feel valued as participants in the early intervention process; at the same time, these skills give service providers a greater sense of satisfaction with their work—all leading to quality services for young children and their families. In closing, it is worthwhile to again remind ourselves of Stephen Covey's (1990) message to seek understanding before seeking to be understood. These words have much to offer early intervention teams.

DISCUSSION QUESTIONS

◆ ◆ ◆   1. You are a service coordinator in an early intervention program responsible for assembling an evaluation team for a new referral. You asked three of your team members from your agency to join the new family's team. During the team's first encounter with the family, it became evident that the values of one of your team members clashes with the family's values. What are some of the potential conflicts, and what are some options for dealing with them if they arise?

2. You just walked out of a team meeting feeling frustrated because you had something really important you wanted to discuss with your team and did not. You tried three times to speak up about your con-

cern; however, no one responded. What steps might you take to ensure that you have a chance to be heard next time the team meets?
Think about strategies you can employ before and during the meeting. If you are not heard in the near future, what do you foresee as
the possible consequences for your team?

3. Your agency's team is relatively stable even though members change
    somewhat with each family's team. Today you learned that your
    agency's team will merge with the team from another agency.
    Describe the implications for team development. What would you
    find most worrisome? What are the positive aspects that could result
    from the change? What are sources of possible discomfort and
    conflict?

4. You are the new leader of a team that is in the performing stage of
    team development. What challenges might you face as the new team
    leader? What leadership style might be effective?

5. Through use of a decision-making process, your early intervention
    team identified a creative response to a family's concern. You, how-
    ever, have to convince your agency administrator to support your
    team's choice, especially since the response does not call for "busi-
    ness as usual" in your agency. What strategies can you use to con-
    vince your administrator? What will you tell her about your team
    process? What will you do if she doesn't support your team's deci-
    sion? What are the implications for the team?

6. Suppose it is your turn to lead an early intervention team that ro-
    tates leadership every 2 months. In the past, every time you facili-
    tated a meeting, one member monopolized much of the discussion
    time. You noticed this happens with some, but not all, of the facilita-
    tors. Knowing this, what might you do to improve team interactions
    at the next meeting you facilitate? Specifically, how might you re-
    duce the time monopolized by the one team member? ◆

REFERENCES

Bolton, R. (1979). *People skills: How to assert yourself, listen to others, and resolve conflict*. New York: Simon & Schuster.

Brahms, J. (1995, February 4). Trust and respect are the key to great communication. *The Capital Times*, p. 6A.

Briggs, M.H. (1991). Team development: Decision-making for early intervention.
Infant–Toddler Intervention: The Transdisciplinary Journal, 1(1), 1–9.

Bruder, M.B., Lippman, C., Bologna, T., & Derrickson, J. (1991). *Higher Education
Faculty Training Institute Manual*. New York: Mental Retardation Institute of
New York Medical College.

Covey, S. (1990). *The seven habits of highly effective people: Powerful lessons in personal
change*. New York: Simon & Schuster.

Dean of Students Office. (1991). *Communication skills trainer's manual*. Madison:
University of Wisconsin–Madison, Dean of Students Office.

Edelman, L., Greenland, B., & Mills, B.L. (1992). *Family-centered communication
skills*. St. Paul, MN: Pathfinder Resources.

Handley, E.E., & Spencer, P.E. (1986). *Decision-making for early services: A team approach.* Elk Grove, IL: American Academy of Pediatrics.

Harry, B. (1992). Developing cultural self-awareness: The first steps in values clarification for early interventionists. *Topics in Early Childhood Education, 12*(3), 333–350.

Herman, P. (assisted by Murphy, M.) (1990). *Parent involvement resource manual: Comprehensive materials for teaching parent involvement.* Madison: Wisconsin Council on Developmental Disabilities.

Hicks, R., & Bone, D. (1990). *Self-managing teams: Creating and maintaining self-managed work groups.* Menlo Park, CA: Crisp Publications.

Individuals with Disabilities Education Act (IDEA) of 1990, PL 101-476. (October 30, 1990). Title 20, U.S.C. 1400 et eq: *U.S. Statutes at Large, 104,* 1103–1151.

Kilgo, J.J., Clarke, B.A., & Cox, A. (Eds.). (1990). *Interdisciplinary infant and family services training: A professional training model.* Richmond: Virginia Institute for Developmental Disabilities.

Kindler, H.S. (1988). *Managing disagreement constructively.* Los Altos, CA: Crisp Publications.

Kolb, D. (1985). *Learning Style Inventory: Self-scoring inventory, and interpretation booklet.* Boston: McBer & Co.

Landerholm, E. (1990). The transdisciplinary team approach in infant intervention programs. *Teaching Exceptional Children, 22*(2), 66–70.

Locke, D.C. (1992). *Increasing multicultural understanding: A comprehensive model.* Newbury Park, NJ: Sage Publications.

Maddux, R.B. (1988). *Team building: An exercise in leadership.* Los Altos, CA: Crisp Publications.

Mealy, D.H. (1984). *Effective team building for managers.* New York: American Management Association.

Menninger, J., & Dugan, E. (1988). *Make your mind work for you.* Emmaus, PA: Rodale Press.

Miller, D.W. (1991). *Strategies for getting teams unstuck.* Potomac, MD: Phoenix International.

Meyers-Briggs, I., & Briggs, P. (1980). *Gifts differing.* Palo Alto, CA: Consulting Psychologists Press.

Nash, J.K. (1990). Public Law 99-457: Facilitating family participation on the multidisciplinary team. *Journal of Early Intervention, 14*(4), 318–326.

Orelove, F.P., & Sobsey, D. (1991). *Educating children with multiple disabilities: A transdisciplinary approach* (2nd ed.). Baltimore: Paul H. Brookes Publishing Co.

Quick, T.L. (1992). *Successful team building.* New York: American Management Association.

Rees, F. (1991). *How to lead work teams: Facilitation skills.* San Diego: Pfeiffer & Co.

Scholtes, P.R. (1988). *The team handbook: How to use teams to improve quality.* Madison, WI: Joiner Associates.

Simons, G. (1989). *Working together: How to become more effective in a multicultural organization.* Los Altos, CA: Crisp Publications.

SkillPath, Inc. (1991). *Coaching and teambuilding skills.* Mission, KS: Author.

Spencer, P.A., & Coye, R.W. (1988). Project BRIDGE: A team approach to decision-making for early services. *Infants and Young Children, 1,* 82–92.

Swan, W.W., & Morgan, J.L. (1993). *Collaborating for comprehensive services for young children and their families: The local interagency coordinating council.* Baltimore: Paul H. Brookes Publishing Co.

Tuckman, B.W. (1965). Developmental sequence in small groups. *Psychological Bulletin, 63,* 385–399.

Wolfe, B.L., Petty, V.G., & McNellis, K. (1990). *Special training for special needs.* New York: Allyn & Bacon.

Zemke, R. (1993). In search of good ideas. *Training Magazine, 30*(1), 46–51.

7

INTERAGENCY COLLABORATION
What, Why, and with Whom?

George S. Jesien

◆ ◆ ◆

OBJECTIVES

◆ ◆ ◆ By completing this chapter, the reader will

- Understand the definition of collaboration and how it differs from co-ordination and cooperation
- Understand the benefits and challenges involved in collaborating with families and other agencies and programs
- Become familiar with elements that foster, as well as elements that hinder, true collaboration among agencies or between service providers and families ◆

What does it mean to collaborate? The *American Heritage Dictionary* (1985) lists two definitions. The first is to "work together, especially in a joint intellectual effort" (p. 291). The second is to "cooperate treasonably, as with an enemy occupying one's country" (p. 291). This second definition suggests the turf issues or agency territoriality that give collaboration a negative connotation in some agencies. Too much collaboration can be seen as disloyalty to one's own profession, program, agency, or organization. In many contexts, however, the term has lost this negative connotation and has in some cases become a buzzword.

In the social services field and particularly in early intervention, the term *collaboration* is used frequently but is not always well defined. Kagan (1991) provided a useful description of collaboration that is used in this chapter. Collaboration is the sharing of power, information, and resources between at least two persons, programs, or agencies to facilitate a mutually beneficial activity or further the achievement of a mutually beneficial goal.

Collaboration has become a foundational concept in early intervention. Peterson (1991) observed that collaboration serves as a basis for conceptualizing the array of services that is needed to provide comprehensive services for young children and their families. An understanding of collaboration and ways to facilitate it will become increasingly important to early intervention service providers and service coordinators as they work with parents and staff from multiple agencies and programs in coordinating services with and for families (Hausslein, Kaufmann, & Hurth, 1992).

Complex problems can be addressed more effectively when programs and agencies coordinate their work to support families. Fragmentation of services results in a multitude of eligibility criteria, application forms, and organizational structures. Learning how such "nonsystems" work is one of the greatest challenges facing families, service coordinators, and service providers. As the Rileys' story in this chapter demonstrates, this challenge often can lead to frustration because seemingly straightforward needs involve such complicated processes. These processes seem most complicated when organizational responsibilities overlap and the need for collaboration is most acute.

Yet, few service providers have received formal training on how to work collaboratively. Although service providers are expected to be capable of a range of collaborative activities, little instruction is provided in most professional training programs (Bruder, Brinkerhoff, & Spence, 1991). Most service providers must learn the intricacies of collaboration on the job as they attempt to establish agreements and working relationships with agencies, other service providers, and parents.

Misconceptions about collaboration—what it is, for whom it is done, and why it is done—hamper intervention efforts and produce less-than-optimal results for children and families. Because the early intervention systems being developed in many states are still "works in progress," early intervention service providers have opportunities to enhance, rejuvenate, and, in some instances, create portions of those systems. An understanding of collaboration will help service providers to use such opportunities to develop systems that are responsive and flexible as well as efficient.

THE RILEY STORY

Tom and Mary Riley need to find a way to pay for a hydraulic lift for their van because their daughter, Tracey, uses a motorized wheelchair. Until now, they have either lifted Tracey and her wheelchair into the van or used a makeshift wooden ramp. As Tracey has grown older and her weight has increased, however, Tom and Mary find themselves hesitating at the difficulty of lifting her into the van for routine shopping trips and family outings.

A friend told them that the county might provide financial help to refit their van with a hydraulic lift. Mary telephoned the county and was referred to a county social services worker. The social services worker asked about the Rileys' income and about whether they were having any family problems. She told Mary that their income was a little too high to qualify for Social Security benefits. She also said that her office did not handle equipment requests, but she thought the local hospital might be able to help.

The hospital suggested calling the state rehabilitation agency in the state's capital. Mary's long-distance call to that agency resulted in her having four more people to call and a host of questions to answer. The last of the four people suggested that Mary call the local family support coordinator—in the county social services agency!

The Rileys are feeling frustrated and angry. They know that their request is neither unheard of nor unreasonable, yet they are beginning to wonder whether it will be possible for them to get what they need.

NEED FOR COLLABORATION

Some of the Rileys' problems could have been avoided if the agencies involved had collaborated with one another to reduce unnecessary duplication and complexity and simplify the procedures for obtaining services. A service coordinator might have facilitated such collaboration.

Children and families have many types of needs: social, economic, physical, educational, and emotional. A family's needs comprise an interconnected web that is not divided easily into separate parts (Bailey, 1989). But supports to meet families' needs are too often organized with rigid boundaries that are usually related to funding sources, bureaucratic relationships, and disciplinary traditions. For example, eligibility for the Medical Assistance Fund (Title XIX of the Social Security Act of 1981, PL 97-35) may be determined by income level only, without regard for the proportion of family income that is spent on needed services. As another example, school districts may focus only on a child's educational needs, overlooking important medical concerns or family needs.

Separate eligibility criteria are used to determine who receives support from various funding sources. These criteria have no relationship to one another. Therefore, some families are eligible for more than one type of assistance, whereas others with similar needs are not eligible for any support. Thus, the system, if it can be called that, often fails because programs are 1) primarily crisis oriented, 2) too categorical in nature to address broad needs, or 3) ineffective because they lack the necessary lines of communication to create coherent efforts with a comprehensive view of families' needs (Melaville & Blank, 1991). The Rileys' experience is typical of that of many families who feel they merely get transferred from one person to another as they try to address their needs for information or resources.

Many families need assistance from more than one source to address their multiple needs. Some struggle to put together a workable package of services. Kochanek (1992) noted that although some families receive multiple services concurrently, others receive no services because they are not identified, do not meet eligibility criteria, or are placed on long waiting lists. Some families become frustrated and abandon their attempts to figure out how to get their needs met in such a fragmented system.

With true collaboration, more families' needs could be addressed with less frustration for service providers as well as families. Collaboration between families and service providers can help services to become more responsive to families and ultimately more effective. Collaboration among agencies would allow service providers to be more efficient and flexible by eliminating unnecessary duplication and by developing compatible entry and service procedures. In addition, through collaboration, a more comprehensive analysis of the challenges faced by families and of opportunities for solutions or supports could be identified (Gray, 1989). Collaboration can result in more coherent, more easily accessible services that can have a great impact on an entire community as well as a synergistic effect on the participating partners (Elder & Magrab, 1980; Mattessich & Monsey, 1993).

Definitions

Terms such as *cooperation* and *coordination* often are used interchangeably with *collaboration,* but each in fact has a distinct meaning. Kagan (1991) presented the concepts of cooperation, coordination, and collaboration as constituting a hierarchical progression that moves toward more sophisticated and complex relationships and that leads to more effective problem solving.

Cooperation

Kagan (1991) described cooperation as individuals or agencies working more or less autonomously but with knowledge of each other's programs and efforts. She views cooperation as forming the base for more complex relationships and sees it as the most prevalent and informal type of relationship. Swan and Morgan (1993) typify cooperative arrangements as agencies that are "autonomous, function independently in parallel fashion and work toward the identified goals of their respective programs" (p. 21). Examples of cooperative activities are the exchange of newsletters, sharing information on procedures and resources, or informally meeting to stay informed of recent developments.

Coordination

With coordination, agencies give up some autonomy to gain certain benefits. Some integration of activities takes the place of only parallel opera-

tions. Coordination often involves agencies modifying the way they operate and is seen by many as a prerequisite for collaboration (Hord, 1986;
Kagan, 1991; Swan & Morgan, 1993). Coordination among agencies and
individuals helps to avoid duplication of efforts and ensures that as many
families as possible are served. Examples of coordination include agencies
joining to conduct a child development screening in the same location on
the same date or agencies consulting with each other to avoid conflicts
when scheduling events.

Collaboration

Resources, power, information, and authority are shared in collabora-
tions. "People work together to achieve common goals that could not be
accomplished by a single individual or agency working independently—
or, at least, could not be accomplished as efficiently" (Kagan, 1991, p. 3).
Bruner (1991) described collaboration as being a means to an end but
not an end in itself. In early intervention, the end is more comprehensive, with appropriate services that improve outcomes for families
(Bruner, 1991).

ACTIVITY: *Organizational Charts*

◆ ◆ ◆   Develop organizational charts for two agencies working at either a local
or a state level. Show graphically and verbally how the two agencies
have overlapping or complementary responsibilities, services, or capabilities. Show the contacts that staff have with one another and with their
service or consumer populations. Indicate any efforts on which the two
agencies do or could cooperate, coordinate, or collaborate. Discuss how
these efforts would change as the agencies evolved from merely coordinating to cooperating and collaborating. What closer working relationships could be developed, and what would be the benefits of such
relationships? ◆

When Is Collaboration Useful?

Because collaboration is a means, not an end, it is not necessary or useful to collaborate in everything. There are situations in which collaborative efforts are particularly valuable, however. Examples include the
following:

• When needs are complex, long lasting, and sustained and shared efforts are needed to address them
• When solutions are not immediately evident or change over time
• When needed improvements in services will require systemic solutions or modifications rather than specific program modifications

- When others have expertise, resources, or relationships that would be helpful in addressing problems

All of these situations exist in many early intervention programs. Families' needs are often complex and long lasting. The needs of a child with disabilities can interact with and affect the needs of other family members and the functioning of the entire family system (Turnbull, Turnbull, Shank, & Leal, 1995). Needs and potential solutions change as the child grows and the family adapts and learns. Needs also can change dramatically when crises occur (e.g., hospitalizations, sudden changes in income, increased demands on financial resources) (Bailey, 1989).

Effective service delivery requires the continuous work of all those involved to maintain flexibility as well as to identify gaps in services. Problems that arise often will require that multiple attempts be made to develop and implement solutions. Thus, a family receiving early intervention services potentially has much to gain from increased collaboration among service providers and families in developing a more comprehensive, coordinated, and flexible system of supports and services.

LEVELS OF INTERAGENCY COOPERATION AND COLLABORATION

Collaboration can occur at several programmatic and organizational levels and will vary in character depending on the context. Collaboration at one level can stimulate collaboration at other levels. Thus, although true collaboration at all levels may seem to be a rather lofty goal, service providers can start at any level, knowing that their efforts will have an impact on those with whom they interact.

Bruner (1991) provided a useful way to conceptualize different levels of collaboration. The levels are 1) collaboration between a service provider and a family, 2) intra-agency collaboration, 3) interagency service-level collaboration, and 4) interagency administrative-level collaboration. Each is described in the subsections following.

Collaboration Between a Service Provider and a Family

Successful collaboration between a service provider and a family is based on mutual information sharing, access to resources, and decision-making power. Both parties, but especially the service provider, need to be honest and straightforward in exchanging information. Families may hesitate to share information until they are sure that its use will not be detrimental. Trust develops over time as a family receives complete and accurate information from the service provider.

Development of a collaborative partnership also requires that both parties have a say in how resources are allocated. If the service provider alone decides which and how often services will be provided, true collaboration will be difficult to establish. Parents need to know that they have

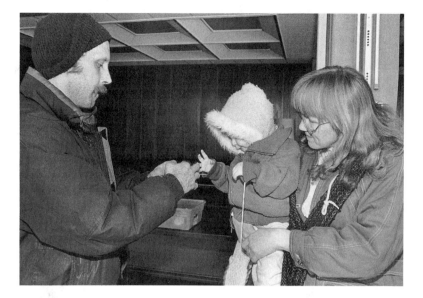

a real say in the services that are delivered, as well as in how and when they are delivered. Conversely, the service provider needs to share fully his or her expertise and professional experience during the decision-making process.

The sharing of power usually requires that each party relinquish some control. For this to happen, each must trust that the decision-making power that is relinquished will be used to achieve mutually agreed-upon goals.

The collaborative relationship between a service provider and a family is based on the understanding that each has something that the other needs. The service provider has knowledge gained from extensive study, practice under expert supervision, and experience with many children and families. Family members have unique and extensive knowledge of the child: his or her strengths, needs, tolerance, characteristics, and approach to challenges. Family members also know what they want and are willing to work toward.

This balance of power usually is skewed in favor of the family because the family can decide how they want to participate in the decision-making process. This point was made by a parent in a class of service providers and parents: "We as a family can succeed without the professional, but the professional always needs the family to succeed in an early intervention program."

Mutual respect for individual values, beliefs, and styles of work and coping are essential to a collaborative relationship. Each person needs to be confident that the others are doing their best. Having confidence in one another allows partners to develop new abilities and resources to face the challenges ahead.

Intra-agency Collaboration

With intra-agency collaboration, staff collaborate with other staff, managers, and administrators within an agency. The degree to which staff collaborate with their colleagues, and the degree to which programmatic and organizational decisions are made in a collaborative manner, are likely to be related to the degree to which staff are willing to collaborate with families. If an agency's structure is hierarchical, with little responsibility and decision-making power shared across staff levels, it is unlikely that a service provider will feel free to seek innovative solutions with a family, or be willing to share decision-making power with them. A collaborative atmosphere among staff at various organizational levels is more likely to lead to collaboration between service providers and families. Too much structure and rigid rules within an agency are likely to give a higher priority to administrative procedures than to families' unique needs.

A collaborative spirit in an agency is often enhanced when staff represent the diverse cultures and backgrounds of the families served by that agency. Hiring parents as full members of service teams increases diversity and ensures that a family perspective is represented on an equal footing with the perspectives of staff members from the various disciplines. Valuing family members as employees can help to foster collaborative relationships within the agency, with the families served, and with the community-at-large (see Chapter 8).

Interagency Service-Level Collaboration

With interagency service-level collaboration, service providers from different agencies work together to provide comprehensive early intervention services. The service providers may have different functions (e.g., screening, evaluation, therapy, service coordination), or they may have similar functions (e.g., providing therapy) while working together so that their services are consistent and mutually supportive. Administrative support is essential at this level of collaboration, as are mechanisms for sharing information. Sharing resources or funding may be necessary, and interagency agreements sometimes are needed concerning issues such as application procedures, eligibility, forms, and evaluation.

Each service provider assumes some responsibility for developing and nurturing effective working relationships with service providers from other agencies. As with collaboration at other levels, these relationships are sustained by sharing information, resources, and decision-making power.

ACTIVITY: *Interagency Agreements*

◆ ◆ ◆   Identify and fulfill a need in your community. Possibilities include the following: developing a coordinated identification system, establishing a single point of referral, developing a resource directory, eliminating duplication of evaluation efforts, and getting additional therapy services. Develop a detailed outline for an interagency agreement for two agencies to use in addressing the need. Be sure to specify the who's and how's of the agreement and the responsibilities of each party. List potential obstacles to drafting and implementing the agreement and possible ways of overcoming these obstacles so that the two agencies move closer to addressing the need collaboratively. ◆

Interagency Administrative-Level Collaboration

Decisions made at the administrative or policy-making level can either foster or hinder collaboration. For collaboration to work at this level, administrators need to recognize that children and families do not belong to their agency or to any other agency. Labels such as "our children" and "your families" indicate a misconception of a service agency's purpose. Children belong to their families, and families belong to their communities.

Administrators can support interagency collaboration by providing permission and incentives for staff at various levels to establish relationships with their counterparts in other agencies. As contacts and exchanges become more frequent, opportunities for collaboration increase.

For interagency collaboration to flourish, the structures of participating agencies need to be flexible enough to change and evolve. In fact, interagency collaboration often alters the structures and functions of participating agencies. Interagency teams can take advantage of creative strategies and mechanisms in addressing common problems. Discussions across agencies often lead to unforeseen procedures, programs, and structures. To embark on a collaborative venture is to introduce an element of uncertainty as new solutions are developed and tried.

ELEMENTS THAT SHAPE
INTERAGENCY EFFORTS TOWARD COLLABORATION

Many characteristics of an agency affect its openness to collaboration. Some of the more important characteristics are discussed in this section.

Social and Political Climate

An agency may be especially open to collaboration when change is occurring. Blank and Lombardi (1992) pointed out that the necessity for change can become apparent when new problems are not addressed adequately, challenges to existing funding or structures arise, new resources become available, new legislation or mandates affect the agency, or a proactive and vocal advocacy constituency voices its concerns.

Communication Process

Collaboration is most likely to succeed when a goal is supported by the consensus of those involved. Some agreement on how to achieve the goal on local and practical levels should be emerging. The extent of collaboration will be determined, in part, by 1) the extent to which participants agree on broad goals and specific steps for implementation, and 2) the degree to which participants are able to maintain frequent and effective communication. The use of open and direct communication can lead to increased trust and support among agency staff (Elder & Magrab, 1980). Communication has been found to be one of the most important elements of effective collaboration (Harrison, Lynch, Rosander, & Borton, 1990).

Leadership and Participation

Effective leadership guides participants through the many possible snags on the way to consensus. Effective leadership facilitates the provision of a forum in which different parties can share their views without causing animosity and meaningful resolution can be achieved through mutual respect and agreement ("Building Interagency Teams," 1990). Swan and Morgan (1993) pointed out that effective leadership can help collaborating parties to develop a vision that can be shared by all.

Leadership encourages the participation of as many "stakeholders" as possible. This increases the likelihood of parents and staff "buying in" to collaborative goals and plans. Good participation also gives a collaborative effort credibility in the community and increases the possibility for widespread support.

Staff Selection, Support, and Training

Change can be difficult. Collaborative efforts alter the roles that individuals traditionally play and may require that individuals modify their attitudes or acquire additional skills as well. New staff who are willing to take on new roles and to explore responsibilities different from those they have had in the past can help in building a flexible and creative team. Often the additional demands on existing staff can be seen as overwhelming if staff members already perceive themselves as being overburdened.

Obtaining staff support for a collaborative venture is critical. It can be developed and enhanced by allowing staff to participate on a voluntary basis, by soliciting their ideas for ways to improve agencies and their effectiveness, and by providing training and staff development activities.

Flexible Policies

Each agency brings its own rules and procedures to a collaborative effort. For collaboration to succeed, an agency must be willing to adapt or change its established procedures to mesh better with those of other agencies or to respond better to the needs at hand. An agency's strict adherence to its own policies and procedures can hinder, if not endanger, a collaborative effort.

Allocation of Resources

Two aspects of resource allocation are important for collaboration. The first is an agency's willingness to share resources to achieve a common goal. This can involve joint funding, sharing the costs of maintaining certain personnel, or combining revenues for a particular purpose.

The second important aspect of resource allocation is the joint pursuit of additional resources from local, state, or federal sources. Extra resources may be very helpful in beginning a collaborative effort (Harrison et al., 1990). It is essential that all parties see themselves as benefiting from and moving closer to a mutually agreed-upon goal.

OBSTACLES TO COLLABORATION

People who initiate collaborative efforts routinely face many obstacles at various levels (Melaville, Blank, & Asayesh, 1993). Most parents, service providers, and administrators could list many obstacles based on their personal experiences. The Riley family mentioned earlier ran into their share of obstacles, many of which were caused by lack of collaboration among agencies and lack of knowledge of those employed by the various agencies. This section lists some of the more common obstacles to collaboration.

The following are examples of personal obstacles to collaboration:

- Reluctance to give up or share power with other people or agencies
- Resistance to crossing disciplinary boundaries established during professional training
- Reluctance to face issues that challenge personal assumptions
- Discomfort with making decisions individually rather than according to prescribed rules
- Resentment of differences in salaries in the various agencies for seemingly comparable work
- Difficulty in finding the time needed to establish and maintain collaborative efforts

The following are examples of organizational obstacles to collaboration:

- Conflicting rules, regulations, and policies in the various state agencies
- Categorical funding and eligibility requirements
- Different styles of work, definitions of terms, or experiences in serving various groups of people

- Competition for scarce resources
- Political differences among agencies' leaders
- Inadequate traditional criteria to determine success and accountability

Given the number of potential obstacles to collaboration, it is interesting to note that there has been a tremendous increase in the number of collaborative efforts since the mid-1980s. The fragmentation and complexity of a categorical service system has frustrated both the people receiving services as well as professionals working to provide those services (Swan & Morgan, 1993). This frustration, coupled with the inability of categorical and fragmented systems to address the needs of children and families comprehensively, has led to the continuing efforts of policy makers, legislators, parents, and service providers to work together to find solutions that enable communities to address the needs of children and families (Baldwin, Jeffries, Jones, Thorp, & Walsh, 1992).

The experiences of people working toward more effective working relationships provide numerous guidelines for facilitating collaboration (Harrison et al., 1990; Melaville & Blank, 1991). Some of the generally accepted guidelines likely to lead to successful collaboration at various levels are listed below:

- Establish a shared goal or vision. Because motivation will be based on this goal or vision, this may be the most important principle of collaboration.
- Establish and maintain frequent, regular, and accurate communication with the participants involved. The long-term success of a collaborative effort may well depend on the effectiveness and regularity of communications. Whether communications are formalized through documents or maintained through informal exchanges may be less important than having open and frequent communication among participants.
- Involve all key participants in the development of activities. Be sure to include those who could contribute as well as those who could pose challenges. Representatives of all the groups that may be affected should also be included. Building ownership at all levels, although time consuming, will maintain a broad base of support.
- Be realistic. Cooperation may be a first step in developing a trusting relationship before true collaboration occurs. Take a developmental approach, and use successes to build closer working relationships.
- Agree to disagree. Total agreement on everything is neither possible nor necessary. Collaboration involves give-and-take on many specific issues. Each party needs to be willing to give in at times to the needs of the others.
- Make realistic commitments. A good strategy is to underpromise and overproduce, especially if participants have experienced previous

failures or frustrations. One small success is often preferable to a
dozen stalled attempts at major change.

- Keep the goal clear. This is especially important when the effort gets
bogged down in administrative details or obstructive regulations.
Keeping the larger vision in the forefront can help in dealing with minor problems, thereby freeing energies for more important tasks.
- Make successes public. They can build momentum for larger systematic changes in programs and agencies. Disseminating information
about successful changes can encourage others to initiate similar efforts or to join in communitywide efforts.

PERSONAL BEHAVIORS AND ATTITUDES
THAT FACILITATE COLLABORATIVE EFFORTS

The heart of collaboration is individuals working together (Bruner,
1991). Regardless of the larger context, everyone can either foster or hinder collaboration in his or her day-to-day contacts with others, whether
parent, professional colleague, or staff from other agencies or programs.
Repeated contacts among staff from various agencies have a cumulative
impact on the willingness of agencies and individuals to enter into collaborative relationships. The following are some suggestions that are likely
to increase the potential for collaboration when working with families
and other service providers:

- Be willing to listen to and understand the needs, goals, and proce-
dures of others.
- Respect the operating procedures of other individuals and agencies.
- Keep the goal in mind.
- Be flexible enough to try many options in working to achieve the goal.
- Be willing to relinquish some decision-making power.
- Be the first to share a resource, assist in an activity, or try a different
way.
- Let someone else take the lead in initiating an activity.
- Give others credit for having accomplished an objective or achieved
success.
- Reach out to a counterpart in another agency. Invite him or her to
participate in an upcoming activity or planning session.
- Do not take others' delays in responding personally. Many people
struggle to get as much accomplished as possible, and some tasks are
bound to slip through the cracks.

ACTIVITY: *Solving the Puzzle*

◆ ◆ ◆   Divide into small groups of five or six people each. Distribute puzzles,
and instruct each group to complete a puzzle without speaking. (Be sure

that each group's puzzle is missing one piece that is in the possession of another group.) Observe how the groups go about solving the problem. Invariably, someone will either speak or go to another group to find the piece missing from his or her group's puzzle.

Ask the participants what they felt while they were doing the task. They are likely to conclude that in order to solve some problems, it may be necessary to bend the rules or not follow standard procedures.

SUMMARY

Collaboration is not a simple solution to the problems that face service providers and their agencies. It is, however, a part of the solution. Collaboration requires the thoughtful efforts of professionals and parents at all levels of service systems—local, state, and national. Greater collaboration certainly would have helped the Riley family as they tried to satisfy a need. Greater collaboration among agency personnel and families will help service systems to be more flexible and responsive in developing novel and creative solutions to the problems that face families and service providers each day.

DISCUSSION QUESTIONS

1. What are the differences among coordination, cooperation, and collaboration?
2. Why is it increasingly important for agencies as well as families and service providers to collaborate in providing early intervention services?
3. What are the factors that facilitate collaboration? What factors hinder collaboration?
4. What behaviors have you observed recently in yourself or in a colleague that could hinder the potential development of a collaborative relationship? What could you do differently to support collaboration?

REFERENCES

American Heritage Dictionary (2nd college ed.). (1985). Boston: Houghton Mifflin.

Bailey, D. (1989). Case management in early intervention. *Journal of Early Intervention, 13,* 87–102.

Baldwin, D.S., Jeffries, G.W., Jones, V.H., Thorp, E.K., & Walsh, S.A. (1992). Collaborative systems design for Part H of IDEA. *Infants and Young Children, 5*(1), 12–20.

Blank, M.J., & Lombardi, J. (1992). *Toward improved services for children and families: Forging new relationships through collaboration.* Washington, DC: Institute for Educational Leadership.

Bruder, M.B., Brinkerhoff, J., & Spence, K. (1991). Meeting personnel needs of PL 99-457: A model interdisciplinary institute for infant specialists. *Teacher Education and Special Education, 14*(2), 77–87.

Bruner, C. (1991). *Thinking collaboratively: Ten questions and answers to help policy makers improve children's services.* Oak Brook, IL: North Central Regional Educational Laboratory.

Building interagency teams. (1990). Tallahassee, FL: Bureau of Education for Exceptional Children, Department of Education.

Elder, J.O., & Magrab, P.R. (1980). *Coordinating services to handicapped children: A handbook for interagency collaboration.* Baltimore: Paul H. Brookes Publishing Co.

Gray, B. (1989). *Collaborating.* San Francisco: Jossey-Bass.

Harrison, P.J., Lynch, E.W., Rosander, K., & Borton, W. (1990). Determining success in interagency collaboration: An evaluation of processes and behaviors. *Infants and Young Children, 3*(1), 69–78.

Hausslein, E., Kaufmann, R., & Hurth, J. (1992, February). From case management to service coordination: Families, policy making, and Part H. *Zero to Three, 12*(3), 10–12.

Hord, S.M. (1986). A synthesis of research on organizational collaboration. *Educational Leadership, 43*(5), 22–26.

Kagan, S.L. (1991). *United we stand: Collaboration for child care and early education services.* New York: Teachers College Press.

Kochanek, T.K. (1992). Federal policy in health and education as a stimulant for a comprehensive early intervention system: Myth or reality. In J.J. Gallagher & P.K. Fullagar (Eds.), *The coordination of health and other services for infants and toddlers with disabilities: The conundrum of parallel systems* (pp. 33–50). Chapel Hill: University of North Carolina at Chapel Hill, Frank Porter Graham Child Development Center.

Mattessich, P.W., & Monsey, B.R. (1993). *Collaboration: What makes it work?* St. Paul, MN: Amherst H. Wilder Foundation.

Melaville, A.I., & Blank, M.J. (1991). *What it takes: Structuring interagency partnerships to connect children and families with comprehensive services.* Oak Brook, IL: North Central Regional Educational Laboratory.

Melaville, A.I., Blank, M.J., & Asayesh, G. (1993). *Together we can: A guide for crafting a profamily system of education and human services.* Washington, DC: U.S. Department of Education, Office of Educational Research and Improvement.

Peterson, N.L. (1991). Interagency collaboration under Part H: The key to comprehensive, multidisciplinary, coordinated infant/toddler intervention services. *Journal of Early Intervention, 15*(1), 89–105.

Social Security Act of 1981, PL 97-35, Title 19, U.S.C. 1305.

Swan, W.W., & Morgan, J.L. (1993). *Collaborating for comprehensive services for young children and their families: The local interagency coordinating council.* Baltimore: Paul H. Brookes Publishing Co.

Turnbull, A.P., Turnbull, H.R., Shank, M., & Leal, D. (1995). *Exceptional lives: Special education in today's schools.* Englewood Cliffs, NJ: Prentice Hall.

III

SERVICE COORDINATION ————————————— ◆◆◆

Service coordination in early intervention is a cornerstone of effective individualized family service plans (IFSPs), services, and partnerships between parents and service providers. Service coordination was included in Part H of the Individuals with Disabilities Education Act (IDEA) of 1990 (PL 101-476) to make families' lives easier. The lawmakers and others who advocated including service coordination in IDEA wanted to protect families from being lone navigators in the early intervention system.

The subject of service coordination is a relatively new one for families, and its effectiveness must be watched and evaluated over time. Some families perceive service coordination as vital; others regard it as a mere bandage on a system in need of major surgery. Effective service coordination is contingent on a good match between a family's needs and the services available to them.

As you read the next three chapters, continue to question the function of service coordination and its place in the lives of families with children with disabilities.

8

SERVICE COORDINATION AND MODELS OF COORDINATION

Amy D. Whitehead

◆◆◆

OBJECTIVES

◆◆◆ By completing this chapter, the reader will

- Know the definition of *service coordination* that is in Part H of the Individuals with Disabilities Education Act (IDEA) of 1990, PL 101-476
- Become familiar with other definitions of service coordination
- Be aware of the central role of parents in service coordination
- Become familiar with five models of service coordination ◆

SERVICE COORDINATION AND PART H OF IDEA

It is important for people involved in early intervention to know the legal requirements for service coordination and to understand the changed attitudes toward families that the law reflects. Part H of IDEA requires that each eligible child, and the child's family, must be provided with one service coordinator. Thus, families eligible for early intervention are entitled to service coordination. Service coordination is an active, ongoing process of helping families to meet the support and service needs that they identify. Part H defines service coordination responsibilities, activities, employment, and qualifications.

Individual states will further define Part H as they proceed with its planning and implementation. The nature of service coordination will be shaped in part by the services available to families in particular regions. In addition, individual states will develop their own systems of service coordination for early intervention that will either 1) be created from scratch, or 2) result from the expansion or modification of existing systems. Regardless of the systems that are established, the law requires that service coordination be provided without cost to families.

Service coordination can entail one thing in a medical facility and quite another in a community-based setting. Its definition may vary from county to county and from state to state. Indeed, two similar agencies in the same town may define service coordination differently.

For example, one agency could define service coordination narrowly to include coordination of a single service that that agency offers. By contrast, another agency might define service coordination broadly to include the coordination of all the services that a family is receiving. A person involved in early intervention needs to understand the spectrum of definitions in order to choose or create one appropriate for his or her own situation.

Many parents of children with disabilities take an active role in coordinating services. Although they might qualify to receive professional service coordination, many families choose to coordinate services themselves for a variety of reasons: staff shortages, high family-to-staff ratios, and delays in service delivery, among others.

THE WEBER STORY

Catherine and Jack Weber were living in a rural community when their first child was born. Tragically, Catherine suffered acute infection and died during labor. Sara, a full-term baby, was delivered by cesarean section. She had aspirated meconium, and her oxygen supply was interrupted during Catherine's complicated labor. Sara spent her first 6 weeks in a neonatal intensive care unit in a city 2 hours from the Webers' home. She was referred to early intervention while still in the hospital. During the first few hours of Sara's life, Jack Weber became both a parent and a widower. As he handled the many details of his wife's funeral, he traveled 4 hours round trip each day to visit his daughter, who was slowly gaining medical stability. Shortly thereafter, Jack became a service coordinator.

When Sara finally came home, Jack took her to see Dr. Allan, the pediatrician at the local clinic. Dr. Allan spent a long time with Sara and Jack. She allowed time for questions and explained how the county's early intervention program operated: Dr. Allan drew a single wheel on the bedpaper. In the center she put herself and the Webers; she then drew spokes leading to medical, developmental, and early intervention specialists. She explained that she would be the primary coordinator of services for the Weber family.

During the first year of Sara's life, Dr. Allan coordinated all of Sara's medical evaluations as well as her entry into an early intervention program. Shortly after Sara came home, Jack decided not to return to work despite the loss of income that he would incur. He stayed at home and received public assistance to help take care of Sara.

Jack learned from the early intervention team how to stimulate Sara, how to do Sara's range-of-motion exercises, and how to feed her. Doctors, specialists, early intervention staff, relatives, and friends telephoned every day with questions, and early intervention therapists—alone, in teams, or with students from the university—visited the Weber home frequently.

Although the early intervention program did offer service coordination to Jack, he decided not to use it. He was told that there was only one service coordinator for all 40 families in the early intervention program and that she was spending most of her time with families who were "not able to help themselves." It was explained to Jack that the service coordinator would be able to see him once every month or so unless he had a crisis, in which case he would get priority. The program director acknowledged that this system was not ideal, but he said it was the best that could be done with limited funding for personnel. Jack felt that he was left with no choice but to learn how to coordinate Sara's services himself.

When Sara was 10 months old, Jack joined several other parents in the early intervention program who held regular support group meetings. Group members arranged to meet with people who could help them learn about home health care, financial assistance, respite care, advocacy groups, legislation regarding education, and more. The support group also helped Jack to deal with Catherine's death and to work through his struggles as a single parent.

By the time Sara was approaching her first birthday, Jack's role was expanding beyond the center of the single wheel. Although Dr. Allan remained in the center with regard to medical issues, Jack now began to occupy the center of a larger wheel. He had needs and concerns for his family that extended beyond the field of medicine into social services and informal supports. Jack began to view Dr. Allan as an advocate. For example, he asked her if she would: write a letter to the Division of Motor Vehicles authorizing specially designated license plates; fill out a form as part of Sara's Supplemental Security Income (SSI) application process; ask the pharmacist to recognize vitamin D as a medication so that it would cost less; and prescribe home nursing care so that he could return to work.

During Sara's second year, the telephone and doorbell continued to ring. The original service providers were joined by a respite worker, a nurse, a surgeon, a gastroenterologist, staff from the communication systems clinic, and the Social Security Administration.

The configuration of the wheel had changed. Now the Webers alone were in the center, and key service providers coordinated specific areas of Sara's development like smaller, adjunct wheels. A physical therapist began to coordinate orthopedic specialty appointments, and a speech-language pathologist referred Sara to the communication systems clinic.

Dr. Allan monitored the neurological and gastroenterological appointments, and an education specialist coordinated planning for Sara's transition into the public school's early childhood program. Jack had formed close working relationships with these service providers, all of whom cared about Sara. Some of them had become his friends. The wheel ran smoothly, producing a comprehensive, coordinated system of services for Sara and Jack.

Although the system seemed to be functioning well, life still was difficult for Jack. The ongoing adjustment to life without Catherine was painful and lonely. Often he would lose patience with Sara's limitations, and he worried that his frustrations might lead him to harm her physically. Sara's progress was minimal at best, and her almost total inability to hold food down and gain weight made life extremely stressful. Living in the rural countryside had seemed so idyllic before Sara was born, and now it was time consuming and logistically burdensome to travel to the medical center 2 hours away.

The service system seemed to be going the extra mile for Sara and Jack, but Jack wondered where his friends were. The magnitude of change in Jack's life had created an irrevocable gap between him and his friends. Indeed, his only friends after Sara's birth seemed to be service providers.

Finances also were an ongoing concern. Jack often did not have enough money to pay for everything, and he was beginning to go into debt. Such daily, highly personal, private, and emotional challenges were often more difficult to face than were the physical challenges of obtaining services.

By observing service providers and other parents, asking questions, and trying new approaches, Jack learned how to be a service coordinator. Being Sara's service coordinator meant that Jack was quickly becoming an expert regarding Sara and her disability. He learned when to use labels, jargon, and technical terms to get needed information and services. If a service was denied, he knew which telephone numbers to call, what types of letters to write, what things to say, and which allies to enlist. He knew how to follow through until his family's needs were met, and he learned that advocacy is an important part of service coordination.

As Sara approached her third birthday, Jack began to plan for her transition from the early intervention program to the early childhood program. He worked with the early intervention program's education specialist, who helped by making telephone calls and by discussing the subject with all of the other service providers who worked with Sara. Jack attended workshops on educational advocacy. The education specialist helped to coordinate a multidisciplinary team for Sara and arranged several meetings between the staffs of the early intervention program and the early childhood program. She also helped Jack to arrange a visit to the early childhood program.

This advanced planning made it possible for Sara to start attending the early childhood program at the beginning of the school year, even though her third birthday was not until mid-September. The transition went smoothly. People from the early intervention program telephoned Jack periodically and went to observe Sara several times in her new environment.

As the Webers made the transition out of early intervention, their need for service coordination in that area faded and was replaced with the need for service coordination in early childhood. Jack began to see that the cycle of beginning, continuing, and ending would occur over and over throughout his and Sara's lives. He realized that his service coordination was the constant that would hold everything together over time.

SERVICE COORDINATION DEFINED

The case management system that has dominated human services in the United States since the 1970s was developed in response to the deinstitutionalization movement. During the 1970s, thousands of people with disabilities left institutional settings and made their homes in communities all over the United States. Case managers were assigned to ensure successful transitions for these people.

Many of the people leaving institutions had cognitive disabilities and/or mental illness. Most had been in institutions for many years and had never been taught the most basic information about community living. For these reasons, the case management system was designed to help people with very limited abilities to help themselves. The relationship between case manager and consumer was one of helper and receiver (Bailey, 1989). Today, the remnants of this system are especially evident in local human services systems, in which highly specialized service coordinators provide full-time direct services to people with disabilities.[1]

The philosophical shift represented by Part H deliberately broke with the traditional model of case management, a model that presumes dependency and helplessness. Part H replaces case management with a variety of innovative models of service coordination that support the interdependence, independence, capabilities, and decisions of the person and/or family receiving services and are therefore more consistent with the family-centered philosophy of Part H. Whether traditional case management will survive as a distinct option for individuals and/or families

---

[1]The descriptions of the historical model of case management and of the first four models of service coordination described on pages 214–218 of this chapter are adapted by permission from Hurth (1991).

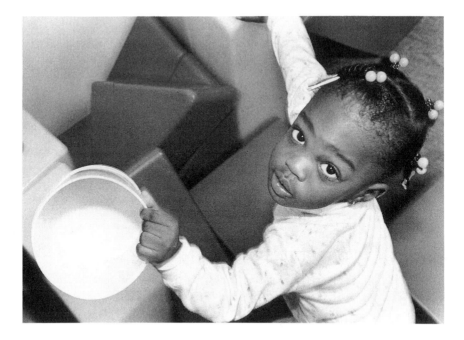

who are literally unable to help themselves remains an unanswered question at this time.

Service Coordination as Defined by Part H of IDEA

Responsibilities

According to Part H, a service coordinator's principal responsibility is to ensure that an eligible child and family receive the early intervention services to which they are entitled. Service coordination is a fluid, proactive process. The service coordinator assists the family in receiving all services identified in the IFSP, coordinates those services, ensures that they are delivered in a timely manner, and seeks additional services that may help the child or family.

Part H lists seven activities for which the service coordinator is responsible:

1. Coordinating the evaluation and assessment
2. Facilitating and participating in the development, review, and evaluation of the IFSP
3. Assisting the family in identifying available services
4. Coordinating and monitoring the delivery of available services
5. Informing the family of the availability of advocacy services
6. Coordinating with medical and health service providers

7. Facilitating the development of a plan for the transition into preschool services, as appropriate

These activities are discussed further in Chapter 9 of this book.

Employment and Assignment

Each state may decide how service coordinators will be employed and assigned within the limits set by Part H of IDEA. Service coordinators must be able to fulfill the responsibilities just listed. (In addition, service coordinators who bill Medicaid are subject to Medicaid employment requirements.)

In Wisconsin, for example, the procedures for employment and assignment of service coordinators vary somewhat from county to county because of the autonomy given to counties in establishing their early intervention programs. In each county, the administrative agency designates a service coordinator for each child referred for evaluation and possible early intervention services. Later in this chapter, several ways in which service coordinators can be employed or assigned are discussed.

Qualifications

According to Part H, service coordinators must understand 1) eligibility requirements for infants and toddlers, 2) Part H and its regulations, and 3) early intervention services and related information in their states. Again, there may be additional requirements for service coordinators who bill Medicaid.

The question of qualifications and competencies is currently under consideration, given Part H's broad definition of service coordinators. Individual states, counties, and programs are working to determine qualifications for service coordinators; in so doing, they may require additional qualifications. In some states, a service coordinator can be any of a number of qualified personnel or a family facilitator who is a parent of a child with disabilities.

The use of unskilled or untrained people as service coordinators is increasingly being explored. Kansas, for example, is investigating this option and has developed a list of competencies of service coordination to define necessary qualifications (Mental Health Services, 1993). These competencies have targeted the following areas of concentration: personal skills development, service coordination, advocacy, content issues, knowledge of developmental milestones, and legal issues (Mental Health Services, 1993).

Some states are utilizing service providers for service coordinator responsibilities, and levels of independence are being divided into distinct categories. In Utah, for example, early intervention personnel are categorized according to credential levels and the corresponding responsibilities and qualifications. The highest credential level is an *early interventionist*

III. These level III personnel are able to perform all service coordinator functions. They must have at least a bachelor's degree (including advanced study), certification or licensure, and 1 year of supervised experience in an early intervention program.

A level II interventionist needs a bachelor's degree and certification or licensure. An early interventionist I requires a high school diploma or a general equivalency diploma (GED) and related training. Although level I personnel may engage in service coordination, it is only under the direct supervision of level II or level III interventionists. Utah also has identified the *early intervention aide* position. A person in this position must have a high school diploma or GED, is supervised by licensed personnel, and has no independent decision-making responsibilities (Striffler, 1993). This model of service coordination allows for both the use of service providers as service coordinators and strict adherence to qualifications standards.

As the issue of qualifications and competencies is explored, levels of autonomy, responsibilities, and tasks must also be addressed (Raiff & Shore, 1993). Service coordinators often need to act independently within a team context. The skilled service coordinator will need to initiate, implement, and follow up on the provision of support to families without constant supervision. These responsibilities often are complex and require a breadth of knowledge about the service delivery system, family dynamics, and interpersonal nurturing. In addition, the tasks involved in service coordination are multifaceted and require a high degree of organization and finesse (Raiff & Shore, 1993). Recommended practice requires that service coordinators be skilled in parent–service provider collaboration, problem solving, and time management.

Terminology and Other Definitions of Service Coordination

Many terms are used to describe the coordination of services. They vary according to discipline and purpose. *Care coordination*, for example, is a medical term that refers specifically to the coordination of a person's medical care. *Service coordination* is more inclusive and refers to health care, human services, and education. Therefore, it is the preferred term in early intervention.

The following paragraphs highlight several definitions of service coordination that differ from or add to the one included in Part H of IDEA:

> The service coordinator assists the family to integrate assessments by health, social/human services, and education professionals and to coordinate and link needed services and funding sources. This process may reduce some duplication of evaluation and service as well as help to determine gaps or service needs that no agency or system is meeting. Service coordination is designed to achieve continuity of optimum, collaborative care by professionals from health, education, and human services systems. (Rosin et al., 1991, pp. 14–15)

"Case management is inherently a simple service—finding out what a family needs and helping them get it" (Morton, 1988, p. 13). For example, if a family identifies as a need the parents having some time alone as a couple, the service coordinator would help them to find respite care: "Family-centered case management refers to services designed to help families locate, access, and coordinate a network of supports that will allow them to live a full life in the community" (Vohs, 1988, p. 41).

The University of Wisconsin's Pulmonary Care Center (1988) pointed out that service coordination must recognize three phases of family need: "initiation, continuation, and reactivation" (p. 25). Most families do not need intensive service coordination every day of their lives. Families can be viewed as being on a continuum in terms of their needs for service coordination. At one extreme is the family in constant crisis or with constant need; at the other extreme is the family who chooses to be completely independent of the service system and opts for no service coordination. Most families fluctuate over time in terms of their levels of need. The service coordinator must be an active listener in order to know when to initiate, continue, or reactivate service.

For example, transitions typically involve increased stress for families. They entail moving from the known to the unknown, and the resultant uncertainty can be difficult. In early intervention, families often form close ties with personnel because their beginnings were with the early intervention program. Leaving early intervention personnel can be emotionally stressful for families. When Sara moves from the early intervention program to the early childhood program, Jack will need to *initiate* relationships with new service providers and a new system. He may choose to *continue* his relationships with Sara's physicians and with his support group. He also may need to *reactivate* some skills he learned when Sara was new to early intervention, such as learning how the human services system is structured, how it is funded, and what laws apply to it.

Parent Involvement

Part H states clearly that parents are primary decision makers in the early intervention process. The right of parents to decide their own levels of involvement in early intervention service coordination is acknowledged. Parents may refuse service coordination altogether, or they might choose to work in close partnership with a service provider to coordinate services.

Empowerment models demonstrate repeatedly that families are more likely to succeed within the human services system if they become involved and acquire skills and knowledge related to service coordination. Involving parents entails treating them with respect and assuming that they have the inherent capacity to make sound decisions concerning their own families (Dunst & Trivette, 1989). Once a parent is involved in the early intervention process, collaboration is possible.

A collaborative relationship between a service coordinator and the parents is the cornerstone of effective service coordination. Trust, honesty, and clear communication in this relationship may encourage parents to participate in early intervention. Because of the importance of this relationship, parents should be involved in choosing their long-term service coordinator. An interim service coordinator may be assigned until the IFSP team determines a long-term service coordinator for the family. Figure 8.1 illustrates the various levels of service delivery and support.

ACTIVITY: *Picturing the Service System*

◆ ◆ ◆   As you understand it, draw a picture of the service system in your area for families who have young children with disabilities. Draw a box to represent each component of the system. Label each box. Add to the picture a circle to represent a family you know whose child receives services from the system. Add lines to show how the family and their service coordinator interact with the service system. Use solid lines to indicate direct contact between the family and the service; use dotted lines to indicate service-to-service contact. ◆

MODELS OF SERVICE COORDINATION IN EARLY INTERVENTION

This section discusses five general models of service coordination. These models were selected to illustrate the range of systems of service coordination possible in early intervention. In all of these models, an interim service coordinator could be used as an initial point of contact for a family until a long-term service coordinator is identified.

Service Coordination Models within Early Intervention Programs

Early intervention programs typically use one of three approaches to coordinating services. There are advantages and disadvantages to each approach. In reading these descriptions, keep in mind that the term *staff person* could refer to a parent hired by a program to coordinate services for families.

Dedicated Service Coordinator

A program using the dedicated service coordinator approach employs one or more staff whose primary or exclusive responsibility is service coordination. The dedicated service coordinator's background may range from service provision to social work. This is the model that was offered

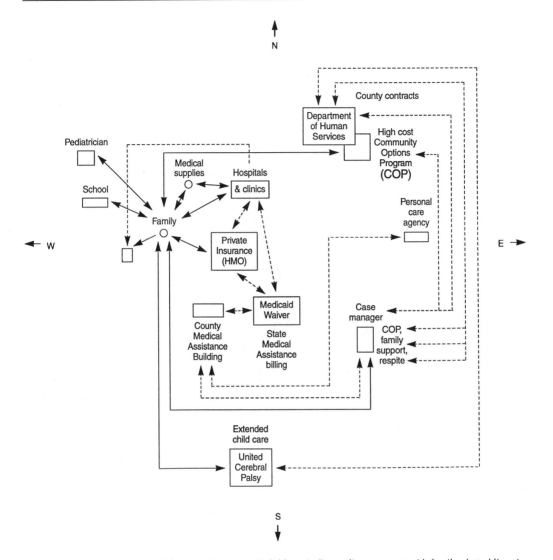

Figure 8.1.   Levels of service delivery and support. (Solid lines indicate direct contact with family; dotted lines indicate state, county, or insurance agency contact only.)

to Jack Weber. In the Webers' story, the program had one service coordinator for all 40 families.

The advantage of the dedicated service coordinator approach is that specific personnel can become highly specialized in one area of expertise. Expertise in building trusting, interpersonal relationships as well as knowledge about the service system potentially make the dedicated service coordinator a highly effective team member. The primary disadvantages of this model are caseload size and the potential for a handful of families to consume all of the service coordinator's time. When caseloads are excessive, the seven activities for which a service coordinator is responsible may be performed minimally for consumers. In addition, with a dedicated service coordinator, there is often less regular contact with the family because weekly appointments may not be scheduled (as they might be for physical therapy, for example).

Most Directly Involved Staff Member

With the most directly involved staff member approach, the staff person who is involved most directly with the family acts as the service coordinator. For example, if a family's greatest needs are related to the child's fine-motor skills, an occupational therapist might be the service coordinator. If the family has complicated issues concerning insurance and SSI eligibility, a social worker could be the service coordinator.

The advantage with this approach is that the frequency of contact between the service coordinator and the family presumably would be higher. In general, a higher frequency of contact should result in a stronger relationship and an increased ability to meet the family's needs. The relative disadvantage is that the staff person most involved with the family may not have any training or detailed knowledge concerning how to work with families or the service delivery system. Traditionally, training for the majority of disciplines related to early intervention has not included information on family issues, interpersonal skills, and/or service delivery.

Individualized Decision

A transdisciplinary team may, through a highly individualized process, decide which staff person would be most appropriate to serve as the service coordinator for a family. This decision takes into account not only the extent of each team member's involvement with the family but also the preferences and interests of family members and staff.

The advantage of this approach is that, in keeping with the intent of Part H, it maximizes individuality and flexibility. The disadvantage is that in programs with a high number of families to serve, the process of decision making may be time consuming and logistically difficult. This approach is most likely to succeed with staff who 1) are committed to the principles of family-centered care, and 2) have strong leaders who can balance staff workloads with individual families' needs.

Community-Level Transagency or Interagency Model

With these models, an interagency team develops a coordinated system for sharing and reviewing referrals. The agency with the greatest involvement in meeting a family's needs is selected to coordinate services for that family.

A four-tier model of service coordination that was developed in a Florida community illustrates interagency collaboration to promote effective service coordination. In the four-tier model, families, physicians, and service providers all have one central point of information and referral (i.e., tier one). Based on preliminary information gathered at this first tier, noncrisis calls are directed to an interim service coordinator (i.e., tier two). The interim service coordinator makes contact with the family as part of the intake process and, when appropriate, the IFSP process is initiated. When early intervention services are necessary, a primary service coordinator is matched with the family (i.e., tier three). Finally, the family is connected with related programs that each have a service coordinator (i.e., tier four). As the service needs of a family become more clearly identified, one of the related program's service coordinators will probably become the primary service coordinator for the family (Cormany, 1993).

The advantage of this model is that areas of specialization exist; therefore, each level of service coordination has a great deal of knowledge and expertise. The disadvantage is that a family might have to readjust continuously to new service coordinators and may never have the time to build relationships at any level. Considering that early intervention is only a 3-year program, and many families enter the program when their children are 1 or 2 years old, this model could contradict the partnerships promised to families in Part H of IDEA.

Consumer and Advocacy Model

With this model, a consumer or advocacy organization is responsible for coordinating services. Such an organization could be part of the formal service system (e.g., through a contract), or it could act independently of the system. Because there is emphasis on consumer empowerment, parents are encouraged to develop their own service coordination skills.

The fact that the service coordinator is outside the early intervention program is both an advantage and a disadvantage of this model. On the one hand, an outside service coordinator may be a stronger advocate because he or she is less tied to the political culture of a particular program. On the other hand, an outside service coordinator may not be as informed on program procedures and may not be included on the early intervention team in the same way as is an in-house service coordinator. For example, when the majority of early intervention staff work in the same program, there are numerous opportunities for them to build relationships that are beneficial for problem solving, information sharing, and overall team functioning. A team member who is not physically on site may have more difficulty in building relationships.

Levels of Service Coordination

Another type of model divides service coordination into state- and local-level functions. For example, a family could have a separate service coordinator for each of the following areas: Medicaid, early intervention, and home health care. This model could incorporate aspects of each of the models discussed previously.

This multilevel model has the same advantages and disadvantages as the community-level transagency or interagency models. Again, the potential exists for highly specialized service coordination within specific areas of expertise. And again, the potential exists for the development of a fragmented service delivery system, with families experiencing numerous and separate applications, contacts, and frustrations.

Coservice Coordination

With the coservice coordination model, parents and a paid professional work together to coordinate services for the family. Often, the family assumes considerable autonomy and calls on the professional as a helpful resource person. This model recognizes that the parents and the professional need one another. The professional probably does not have the time to do intensive service coordination for every family with whom he or she works, so he or she depends on working with a certain number of resourceful families. Similarly, the parent sometimes needs the professional to serve as an advocate or a guide to the ever-changing service delivery system. In order for this model to work, a strong relationship between the parents and the professional is necessary.

The coservice coordination differs from the consumer and advocacy model in that in the former, the family works with a paid professional. In the consumer advocacy model, the family works with an outside organization. Shared responsibility for service coordination entails that parents can "maintain, or come to gain, power over their lives" (Sokoly & Dokecki, 1992, p. 27). Each partner needs skills in collaboration, advocacy, and problem solving. Figure 8.2 delineates this model more clearly. One circle represents the parent, and the other represents the professional. Their independent and shared responsibilities change over time.

Coservice coordination can be a modification of any of the models described here. The paid professional can be employed by an early intervention program, service agency, or advocacy organization. In the past, many parents have volunteered time and energy that surpassed the levels expected of typical parents. With the reauthorization of Part H, there is official recognition of the valuable roles that many parents play in coordinating services for their own children: "A State may, at its discretion, decide as a matter of State policy or practice to pay a parent to be his or

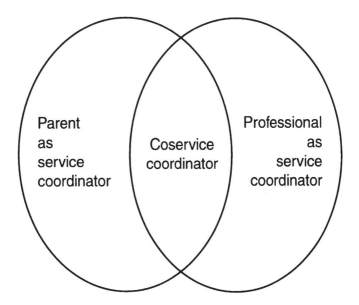

Figure 8.2.   Coservice coordination.

her own service coordinator or reimburse a parent for carrying out certain tasks" (Maroldo, 1991, p. v).

Several pilot projects have provided parents and service providers with an opportunity to learn service coordination skills together. In Colorado, for example, the Mile High Down Syndrome Association organized a 6-month training program for 12 families and their service coordinators. The group met regularly to learn together about family-centered early intervention, with an emphasis on service coordination (Mile High Down Syndrome Association, 1991). One of the positive outcomes of this and similar projects is that parents and service providers are exposed to one another's perspectives, strategies, and strengths. Such an approach to skill building and practice facilitates complete parent–service provider collaboration that is consistent with the intent of Part H.

The coservice coordination model promotes parent empowerment and independence. It allows for the family to play a principal and continuous role in defining their own level of involvement. A caution concerning this model is that some programs could make assumptions about which families are capable of coservice coordination when, in fact, participation should be the family's choice. Another caution is that families could be asked to assume responsibilities that they may not want or be ready for in order to reduce a service coordinator's caseload stress. A final caution involves the issue of payment for services in the event that a family member assumes service coordination responsibilities. This outstanding issue needs further attention and consideration.

ACTIVITY: *The Great Debate*[2]

◆ ◆ ◆   Participants will divide into three groups and be assigned one of the following positions in support of a particular model of service coordination:

Resolved: The service coordinator should be employed by the early intervention program and selected from the discipline most related to the needs of the child and family.

Resolved: The service coordinator should be independent of the early intervention program. He or she should be a "dedicated" service coordinator (i.e., the role is his or her occupation) employed by a separate agency or private provider.

Resolved: The service coordinator should be a parent with experience in raising a child with special needs. Whether the service coordinator is employed by or independent of the early intervention system, he or she should be a parent with special training to assume this role.

The group task is to prepare a position statement outlining the advantages of your model and the comparative disadvantages of your opponents' models. *Remember, this is a debate*; regardless of personal opinions, you must develop a clear argument to support your group's assigned position.

Prepare for the rebuttal round by anticipating the shortcomings your opponents might cite concerning your model and by developing some good counterarguments. Select a spokesperson to represent your group's position in the debate. If two people are selected, divide the responsibilities (e.g., one person could present the position, and the other could present the rebuttal).

Finally, conduct the great debate:

Round 1: Positions are presented. Each speaker or team will have 5 minutes to proclaim the advantages that his or her model has over all the others.

Round 2: Conduct the rebuttals. Each speaker or team will have 5 minutes to challenge the ideas presented by their opponents.

Round 3: Conduct a large group discussion whose purpose is to add other perspectives, to synthesize, and to examine the implications for planning and providing service coordination. ◆

[2]This activity is adapted by permission from Hurth, J. (1991). *Providing case management services under Part H of IDEA: Different approaches to family-centered services coordination.* Chapel Hill, NC: National Early Childhood Technical Assistance System.

EMERGING MODELS OF SERVICE COORDINATION

Service coordination is in its infancy; therefore, its character, shape, strengths, and weaknesses still are largely unknown. Part H intended for service coordination to develop into a positive practice for helping families. It is yet unclear whether service coordination will add another layer of bureaucracy for families or whether it will be the practice that enables families to succeed. Naturally, given the variety of models and approaches to service coordination that exist, both outcomes will probably occur over the next several years or until service coordination is better understood.

SUMMARY

The definitions of service coordination still vary, depending on who is using the term. Part H defines service coordination clearly, and perhaps this definition will influence other areas as well. Currently, states are implementing a variety of models of service coordination, often based on the past functioning of local governments. Early intervention law is intended to facilitate flexibility and individuality—qualities clearly evident in the service coordination that is unfolding.

DISCUSSION QUESTIONS

◆ ◆ ◆

1. To how many separate agencies, programs, or buildings does a family in early intervention relate? To how many individual service providers?

2. What does the map in Figure 8.1 tell you about the responsibilities of the service coordinator? What does it say about the qualifications for service coordinators?

3. What implications does the map in Figure 8.1 have for the provision of family-centered, coordinated care?

4. Write your own definition of service coordination consistent with Part H of IDEA.

5. How might a service coordinator facilitate family-centered care?

6. What qualifications (beyond those required by law) do you think a service coordinator would need to be effective?

7. How could a service coordinator unknowingly build barriers to services?

8. What strengths and weaknesses do you see in each model of service coordination?

9. How might you incorporate more than one model of service coordination into your work as a service coordinator or service provider?

10. How might a particular model of service coordination affect the behavior of a family for whom services are being coordinated? Choose two models and contrast their probable impact on a family.

11. In what situations would coservice coordination be especially effective? ◆

REFERENCES

Bailey, D. (1989). Case management in early intervention. *Journal of Early Intervention, 13,* 120–134.

Cormany, E. (1993). Family-centered service coordination: A four-tier model. *Infants and Young Children, 6*(2), 12–19.

Dunst, C., & Trivette, C. (1989). An enablement and empowerment perspective of case management. *Topics in Early Childhood Special Education, 8,* 87–102.

Hurth, J. (1991). *Providing case management services under Part H of IDEA: Different approaches to family-centered services coordination.* Chapel Hill, NC: National Early Childhood Technical Assistance System.

Individuals with Disabilities Education Act (IDEA) of 1990, PL 101-476. (October 30, 1990). Title 20, U.S.C. 1400 et seq: *U.S. Statutes at Large, 104,* 1103–1151.

Maroldo, R.A. (1991). *Individuals with Disabilities Education Act (IDEA) (as amended by PL 102-119, the Individuals with Disabilities Education Act Amendments of 1991).* Horsham, PA: LRP Publications.

Mental Health Services. (1993). *Proposed service coordinator (case manager) competencies.* Paper developed by the Mental Health and Retardation Services and Family Services Coordination (Case Management) of the Part H State Plan, Topeka, KS.

Mile High Down Syndrome Association. (1991). *Taking charge: Family-centered case management* (Videotape). Littleton, CO: Author.

Morton, D.R. (1988). Case management for early intervention services. *Family Support Bulletin.* Washington, DC: United Cerebral Palsy Associations.

Raiff, N.R., & Shore, B.K. (1993). *Advanced case management.* Beverly Hills: Sage Publications.

Rosin, M., Wuerger, M., Schauls, L., Paisley, R., Sternat, J., & Ditscheit, J. (1991). *Wisconsin ASHA Infant Team Report.* Madison: Wisconsin Personnel Development Project.

Sokoly, M., & Dokecki, P. (1992). Ethical perspectives on family-centered intervention. *Infants and Young Children, 4*(4), 23–32.

Striffler, N. (1993). *Current trends in the use of paraprofessionals in early intervention and preschool services.* Chapel Hill, NC: National Early Childhood Technical Assistance System.

University of Wisconsin, Pulmonary Care Center. (1988). *Seeking effective ways to coordinate care for children with special needs: Wisconsin, Minnesota, and Michigan perspective.* Madison: Author.

Vohs, J.R. (1988). *What families need to know about case management.* Boston: Federation for Children with Special Needs.

9

ROLES OF SERVICE COORDINATION

Amy D. Whitehead

◆ ◆ ◆

OBJECTIVES

◆ ◆ ◆

By completing this chapter, the reader will

- Know the roles, responsibilities, and level of knowledge expected of service coordinators according to Part H of IDEA
- Understand the primary roles of parents in directing and receiving service coordination
- Understand how a service coordinator can be a creative problem solver, advocate, and agent for systems change   ◆

The roles and responsibilities of service coordinators, which are outlined in Part H of the Individuals with Disabilities Education Act (IDEA) of 1990, PL 101-476, need to be understood so that families receive the services to which they are entitled. A service coordinator should be what a family needs him or her to be. The service coordinator must be willing to assume any of a range of roles in response to the varying needs of a family. Practices will be enhanced by careful consideration of the advantages and challenges of these roles.

In addition to helping families directly, service coordination has the potential to improve the service delivery system. A service coordinator is the link between a family and administrators—a voice within the system for the family. By articulating the challenges that face a family, a service coordinator can be an agent for change within the system.

A PROFESSIONAL'S STORY

Anne Bray was driving to an apartment on the south side to visit a family for whom she coordinated services. Anne has had bimonthly visits with the Ross family for over a year now. Anne's training was in occupational therapy, and at first it was difficult for her to expand her range of roles to include service coordination. Now, however, she feels good about her role as a service coordinator.

As she drove along, she reflected on the first time she met the Ross family, which was during the evaluation process. Anne and Helen Ross had had a rocky start. Anne felt that this was primarily because her training had not included family issues, only evaluation and treatment of motor needs. Yet Helen Ross was strong and gave Anne the confidence to function in her new role. They worked together to develop an individualized family service plan (IFSP) for Helen's son John and to ensure that his complex needs were being met with appropriate services. John had severe respiratory problems, a cognitive delay, and hearing loss, and he still lacked a clear diagnosis. Anne offered to provide the family with information on available advocacy services, and she ensured that all of John's health care professionals shared information and reports.

Today, however, something was bothering Anne as she prepared to visit the Ross family. She had just received a copy of a letter from the Social Security Administration stating that John was no longer eligible for Supplemental Security Income (SSI). Anne had helped the family to apply for SSI for John last year; the monthly funds allowed John's mother to work part time and to spend more time with her children. SSI and Medicaid had been the sole sources of health insurance for the family, since the Rosses were divorced. Helen Ross did not have insurance through her job, and her ex-husband, Charlie, was unemployed. Medicaid had been paying for the frequent hospitalizations to treat John's respiratory distress.

Anne parked in the apartment complex lot and walked up to the Rosses' door. Helen Ross answered the door and welcomed her inside. They sat at the kitchen table and Anne showed Helen the letter from Social Security. Helen said she had also received a copy of the letter and that SSI was the least of her worries; she was only concerned with her ex-husband. She said that he had recently come to the apartment under the influence of alcohol and threatened to take the children if Helen did not give up her right to monthly child support. The children were in the room during the altercation. Helen still was visibly shaken from the experience.

Now Anne was faced with the fact that her primary agenda was to assist Helen in appealing Social Security's decision, even though that clearly was not part of Helen's agenda. Anne felt overwhelmed. She had only been out of school for 2 years, and she was herself unmarried and without children. Anne was self-conscious about her youth, inexperience, and "protected" life. She finally remembered to take a breath, shift gears, and listen to Helen. Anne recognized that, at that moment, Helen's overriding concerns were the safety and well-being of her family.

Anne listened and assisted Helen in identifying options to help make her family situation better. Anne asked, "How can I help?" Helen replied, "You can be here for me. Just like you're here for me now." Anne listened further to Helen and asked questions to help structure her options (e.g., "What has been done in the past?", "Do you have a lawyer to address the questions of custody and child support?", "Would you consider filing a complaint or requesting a restraining order?"). Together they developed a plan: Helen would call her lawyer and find out about her legal options. She also would ask her sister, who lived in the same building, to be on-call to take care of the children in case Helen's ex-husband came by again; she could thus try to talk with him without the children present. The plan also included a follow-up call from Anne in a few days.

As Anne left the apartment, she felt a mixture of emotions. On the one hand, she felt frustrated by the complexity of the situation and by her inability to help Helen in a concrete way. For a moment, she wished she were back in a hospital setting in which patients would come to her and occupational therapy would be her major role. On the other hand, she felt reaffirmed in her role as a service coordinator. She had been able to join with the family to meet their immediate needs by putting her own priorities and insecurities aside.

A big question still remained: How could Anne help Helen to realize that the financial burdens would be devastating without SSI and Medicaid? The time line for an SSI appeal meant that Anne would have to act fast; however, Helen was not making this a priority. Anne felt a mixture of conflicting feelings: the need to advocate for John's right to health coverage and the need to respect Helen's priorities. Anne had much thinking to do.

ROLES OF SERVICE COORDINATORS REQUIRED BY PART H OF IDEA

Part H divides service coordination into seven categories. These seven categories describe the activities for which service coordinators in early intervention are responsible.

The Seven Activities

Coordinating Evaluation and Assessment

The service coordinator is responsible for scheduling and coordinating the evaluation and assessment. Working with the family, the service coordinator decides which disciplines should be represented on the early intervention team. In addition, whether to use standardized testing must be decided, and a specific test (e.g., Bayley Scales of Infant Development [2nd ed.] [Bayley, 1993]) must be agreed upon. Depending on family preferences and staff expertise, other testing options may be utilized as well (e.g., a transdisciplinary play-based assessment).

Ensuring that scheduling is convenient for the family also is an important responsibility. A family assessment may be useful for understanding the family, although it must be emphasized that this is voluntary for the family. It is the family who decides what information to share with service providers.

Facilitating and Participating in Development, Review, and Evaluation of the IFSP

The service coordinator, in collaboration with the family, is responsible for all aspects of the IFSP. This responsibility includes 1) scheduling a meeting time for the IFSP team; 2) identifying family concerns, priorities, and resources; 3) providing information about parent rights; 4) developing a written plan and/or working document; and 5) answering any questions that the parents and service providers may have about the process or program. (The IFSP is discussed in detail in Chapter 4 of this book.) In coordinating the IFSP, the parents and service providers join together to explore family priorities and what options are available in light of these (Sokoly & Dokecki, 1992).

Assisting Family in Identifying Available Services

The service coordinator helps the family to identify available services. This includes ensuring that the family knows about all of the available service options. Once the family decides on a service option, the service coordinator must make sure that they obtain that service. This may include assisting the family in obtaining and completing applications (e.g., insurance, public assistance) and helping the family to discuss needs with referral sources (Gilbert, Sciarillo, & Von Rembow, 1992).

In addition to these required services, the service coordinator may help the family to find other resources, such as respite care or informal supports. Informal supports are especially valuable to families regardless of where they live (Whitehead, Brown, & Rosin, 1993). Church organizations, community groups, friends, family, tribes, and other groups can provide emotional support as well as child care, transportation, and problem-solving ideas. Informal supports may last a family's lifetime, whereas the formal supports of the service delivery system continue to change with age, diagnosis, and new legislation.

Coordinating and Monitoring Delivery of Available Services

The service coordinator coordinates and monitors the delivery of services to the family. Once a service is obtained or initiated, monitoring is needed to ensure that it continues to meet the family's needs. For example, it is not enough for a service coordinator to provide a family with information about a Medicaid Waiver program. The service coordinator must follow up to find out if the family needs help with the application, to investigate a denial, or to support the family during annual eligibility reviews. A family may need to switch service providers for a variety of reasons, ranging from a service provider's retirement to parents' dissatisfaction. When a service is continuing but a transition to a new service provider occurs, coordination and monitoring must continue.

Informing the Family of Availability of Advocacy Services

The service coordinator explains to the parents their legal rights within the early intervention system. These rights include the right to appeal decisions with which they disagree and the right to have disputes mediated by a neutral person. The service coordinator also informs the parents of other local, state, and national advocacy resources that may help them to resolve disagreements with early intervention service providers, schools, health care service providers, and other people or systems. Examples of state resources include the following: parent training and information centers, protection and advocacy organizations, and councils on development disabilities. Nationally, there are numerous advocacy organizations for parents, including the National Parent Network on Disabilities as well as many disability-specific organizations (e.g., United Cerebral Palsy Associations). State directories can provide families and service providers with telephone numbers and addresses for these organizations.

In many cases, informing parents of opportunities to connect with other parents also is a function of advocacy. Parent support groups, skill-building workshops, local or national conferences, and parent-to-parent relationships can all enhance parents' levels of confidence, knowledge, and skills.

Coordinating with Medical and Health Service Providers

The service coordinator may coordinate medical and health services. This activity needs to be considered in light of family preferences and circumstances. Many parents would rather arrange for health care services on their own. In some cases, the primary care physician may act as the coordinator for medical services, or a cerebral palsy clinic may handle the arrangements for orthopedic surgery. Because these are routine occurrences, confusion and duplication of efforts would result if the early intervention service coordinator tried to take responsibility. Given the efforts toward national health care reform, ongoing changes will need to be monitored and understood as part of service coordinators' health care coordination.

In the Rosses' story, Anne assisted Helen in obtaining SSI, which included eligibility for Medicaid. Therefore, Anne worked to maintain John's health insurance coverage.

Facilitating Development of a Plan for the Transition into Preschool Services, as Appropriate

The service coordinator coordinates planning for the transition out of early intervention, when appropriate. Transitions are not limited to leaving early intervention. It is important to emphasize that transition planning also should occur when a child leaves a hospital, county, or state, for example.

Times of transition can be extremely stressful for a family and service provider. Often, strong relationships have formed, and changes in relationships (as a result of a transition) may be more difficult for the family than the program transition. (Transition planning is discussed further in Chapter 10 of this book.)

ACTIVITY: *Seven Activities of Service Coordination*

◆ ◆ ◆   Prepare a transparency or worksheet with three column headings: knowledge, skills, and tasks. Divide into small groups and ask each group to look at the seven activities of service coordination. Identify the level of knowledge, skills, and tasks necessary for each activity. Have each small group report its findings to the group as a whole. Facilitate a discussion highlighting the similarities across activities and the level of knowledge and skills that a service coordinator needs. Use Table 9.1 to lead into a discussion of the challenges faced by service coordinators. ◆

Beyond the Seven Activities

The implementation of Part H often has led service coordinators to assume roles that are broader and more complex than those outlined in the

Table 9.1.   Challenges faced by early intervention service coordinators

- Is service coordination a long-term solution or a temporary bandage? Are money and energy spent in maintaining "systems navigators," or does service coordination simplify and improve the system so that consumers can freely gain access to it?
- How will service coordinators provide quality service coordination to each family when they are responsible for so many families?
- How can service coordinators operate on a proactive basis rather than on a respond-to-crisis basis?
- How will service coordinators keep up with the frequent changes in services covered by health care programs and/or eligibility requirements for programs such as Medicaid?
- How can service coordinators share with parents the service coordination skills necessary to maneuver in the system?
- How will service coordinators acknowledge and respect parents who choose 1) to do coservice coordination, or 2) to coordinate services on their own?

Rosin, P., Whitehead, A., Tuchman, L.I., Jesien, G.S., & Begun, A.L. (1993). *Partnerships in early intervention: A training guide on family-centered care, team building and service coordination.* Madison: Waisman Center, University of Wisconsin–Madison; reprinted by permission.

law. Service coordinators daily face challenging situations that call for creative problem solving. They advocate regularly on behalf of families as families struggle to identify ways to finance early intervention services, and many are finding themselves with an opportunity to be agents for systems change. Service coordinators are insiders in the service delivery system. This gives them an opportunity to think critically about the internal strengths and weaknesses of the system.

Challenges

Service coordinators in early intervention daily confront numerous issues ranging from working with families who are struggling to find food, clothing, and shelter to supporting families who have knowledge and expertise that far exceed their own. A service coordinator might be the sole early interventionist working in a rural county with few resources and many miles between agencies and families, or he or she may work in an urban area that offers an array of services, turf issues, and waiting lists, and where there are safety concerns and ethical dilemmas.

An example of a typical challenge in service coordination is the home visit. Part H emphasizes service delivery options for families and encourages the provision of early intervention services in natural environments: "To the maximum extent appropriate, [services] are provided in natural environments, including the home, and community settings in which children without disabilities participate" (Individuals with Disabilities Education Act of 1990, section 1472, [xiv] [G]). In an effort to provide options, many programs offer home visits as well as center-based services. A service coordinator needs knowledge, understanding, and skills to work in either of these environments. Anne, for example, found herself in a position in which she needed to support Helen Ross regarding the issue of an angry, threatening ex-husband. This classic social work issue challenged her training in occupational therapy.

Transportation, child care, and time present logistical barriers for many families. One positive aspect of home visits is that they make services convenient for families (Fallon & Harris, 1992). A service coordinator who provides home-based services (i.e., home visits) will learn about the family in a way that cannot always be possible in a center-based setting. In keeping with the spirit of Part H, the service coordinator has the opportunity to build relationships with the family and learn more quickly about what is meaningful to them.

Some families may, however, perceive home visits as invasive, intrusive, or burdensome. Some families will have had previous associations with human services and social services (e.g., out-of-home placements) involving home visits that were judgmental, laden with assumptions, threatening, and/or demeaning. In addition, some parents may prefer center-based services to get the chance to get out of the house or to network with other parents. A service coordinator and parents can discuss options for where to meet and the relative advantages and disadvantages of various approaches.

At times, service coordinators who conduct home visits may observe family weaknesses that pose ethical dilemmas. Service providers are trained and are required to fully respect the confidentiality of a family. In confidence, a parent may share concerns about his or her child's safety (e.g., issues of physical or sexual abuse[1]) or exposure to inappropriate behaviors (e.g., substance abuse or violence) (Wasik, Bryant, & Lyons, 1990). Confidentiality is crucial for successful service coordination and relationship building, and strong parent–service provider partnerships are needed to find ways to ensure the health and safety of a child and family and to meet the service coordinator's legal obligations. Systems of peer support and/or supervision and mentorship can assist a service provider in making decisions about tough issues of confidentiality (Gilkerson, & Young-Holt, 1992).

ACTIVITY: *Time Management*

◆ ◆ ◆   Imagine that you are the service coordinator for 40 families and that you also have a multitude of administrative responsibilities. What strategies would you use to set priorities and manage your time? How could you give equal time to all families instead of responding only to crises? ◆

Advocating

Service coordinators face advocacy issues when working with families. Several advocacy issues involve financing early intervention services.

Part H of IDEA clearly states that a service coordinator in early intervention looks at the comprehensive needs of the child. One of these needs may be how to finance the child's early intervention services. In the Rosses' story, Anne found herself advocating for the continuation of John's SSI. Her advocacy plan was to work with Helen Ross in filing an appeal.

Studies have documented that early intervention services for children who are at risk can reduce the later need for special education services (Ramey, Bryant, & Suarez, 1990). Knowing that money spent today will decrease future spending, however, has not remedied the financial challenges of early intervention. As more children are identified for early intervention because of Child-Find efforts; decreased stigma; improved public awareness; and increases in prenatal substance abuse, neglect, and exposure to human immunodeficiency virus (HIV) (Zipper, Weil, &

---

[1]In many states, service coordinators are bound by laws that require them to report suspected abuse.

Rounds, 1991), more funding will be necessary to cover the costs of services. States will need to review existing and flexible public and private funding that is available to meet the requirements for implementation of Part H. Medicaid, Chapter 1, Maternal and Child Health Block Grants, and private insurance will be major stakeholders in funding early intervention (Swan & Morgan, 1993). Service coordinators will need to be knowledgeable, resourceful, and creative in learning how, when, and where to gain access to funding.

Acting as Agents for Systems Change

Service coordinators have the potential to initiate significant change. There are many ways in which service coordinators can work to make the early intervention system more accessible and user friendly for families of children with disabilities. Possibilities include the following:

- Organizing parent support, advocacy, or networking groups
- Identifying gaps or areas of duplication within the early intervention system
- Serving on interagency task forces to help integrate the service system's procedures and materials (e.g., consumer satisfaction surveys)
- Working to reduce the number of forms that families must complete and questions they must answer (e.g., by simplifying eligibility criteria or by using common referral and intake forms)
- Participating in training sessions about partnerships between families and service providers, communication skills, health care financing, and other areas related to service coordination

In addition, service coordinators can help to make the early intervention system more accountable by educating parents. Parents who have learned service coordination skills can be powerful agents for systems change. Parents and service providers working together for change combine the outsider's freedom of expression with the insider's knowledge of the system. Their combined efforts are often more effective. Given the range of services available for families, service coordination in early intervention presents some special challenges (see Table 9.1).

ACTIVITY: *A Plan for Change*

◆ ◆ ◆   Identify one service delivery practice or method that is inefficient, wasteful, or non–family-centered. Develop a plan for change. Who would have to "buy in" to your plan in order for it to succeed? How might you persuade them?   ◆

Roles of Parents in Service Coordination

In the Rosses' story, Helen Ross is receiving service coordination from an early intervention program, and she is recognized fully as a primary decision maker on her early intervention team. She collaborated with Anne to develop an IFSP and to arrange services, including financial services (e.g., SSI). In the story, Helen describes and defines how Anne, the service coordinator, can be useful in her particular situation. Her statement, "You can be here for me," reveals that she needs Anne to listen and offer emotional support.

Service coordination was established as a primary component of Part H. It recognizes the need to have one central person who assists a family in making their way through the complex service delivery system. As described in the law, service coordination is a service provided to families. Parents, therefore, have the right to determine their own levels of involvement in the service coordination process.

The roles of parents in service coordination vary, not only from family to family but also from day to day for any one family. For example, during hospitalizations, after new diagnoses, and during transitions, a service coordinator may be needed often by a family. At times when services are being delivered smoothly and no major changes are occurring, however, the service coordinator may be needed less often. In addition, a parent's role often varies, depending on his or her available time. Time is both a resource and a constraint for families of young children (Brotherson & Goldstein, 1992). This fact must be recognized by service coordinators.

There often is a tendency to label parents as "good" or "bad," "easy to work with" or "noncompliant," or "stable" or "dysfunctional." Some families are labeled as "difficult" (Boutte, Keepler, Tyler, & Terry, 1992). Using these sorts of labels creates barriers to collaboration by setting up hierarchical relationships in which professionals presume to be superior to families (Wright & Levac, 1991). Family-centered service coordination is successful when the roles of parents are defined in terms that support rather than demean. Understanding families, behaviors in the contexts of their cultural backgrounds and in light of their life experiences and resources (e.g., time, transportation, education), rather than ascribing derogatory labels to families, leads to family-centered practices.

Parents receiving service coordination during early intervention have a unique opportunity to learn service coordination skills by watching their service coordinator, asking questions, and practicing. Service coordinators should see themselves as guides to the system and should share knowledge and skills with parents. The rate and extent of sharing will be determined by individual parents and service coordinators. For parents, the likely result will be increased independence, control, and self-esteem. This educational process prepares parents for the time when

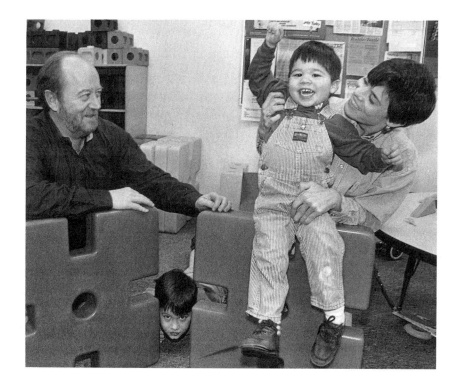

their children leave early intervention and their early intervention service coordinator. Some families will never have another service coordinator; the skills and knowledge gained during early intervention will help them for years to come.

Families, in turn, can teach service coordinators about service coordination in a variety of ways (e.g., Helen Ross's ability to instill Anne with confidence); a family that works within the system can provide inside information on how to gain access to hard-to-find resources.

SUMMARY

The roles of service coordinators are multifaceted and highly varied, and they depend on the situations and the cultural backgrounds of individual families. One service coordinator may have time only to keep up with paperwork, whereas another might have the time to build effective relationships. Many times, different approaches depend less on individual styles of service coordination and more on the structure within which a service coordinator functions.

New roles for service coordinators are continually being created. Training and competencies for these roles are also emerging and vary highly from region to region. Just as early intervention is still taking shape, service coordination will be more clearly defined as time progresses.

DISCUSSION QUESTIONS

◆ ◆ ◆

1. Think of two or three examples of each of the seven activities of service coordinators.
2. Think of an early intervention program with which you are familiar. Who coordinates services for families? If there are gaps in or duplications of services, how might they be avoided? If the usual service coordinator were not available (due to a long illness or layoff), who else could possibly fill the service coordinator role?
3. As a service coordinator, you are approached by a mother who has never met another family with a child having the same disabilities as her daughter. She is eager to meet such a family. How could you help? What would you need to know about the mother's family and about a potential match?
4. How can a service coordinator determine the extent to which parents want to be involved in service coordination?
5. How would a service coordinator go about identifying parts of the system that are not working?
6. Consider the complexity of the service delivery system (local, state, and federal), the efforts toward national health care reform, the limited availability of funding, and the many funding sources that are claiming "payor of last resort." Identify ways in which your state supports services that are family centered, community based, and coordinated. ◆

REFERENCES

Bayley, N. (1993). *Bayley Scales of Infant Development* (2nd ed.). San Antonio: Psychological Corporation.

Boutte, G.S., Keepler, D.L., Tyler, V.S., & Terry, B.Z. (1992, March). Effective techniques for involving "difficult" parents. *Young Children*, 19–22.

Brotherson, M.J., Goldstein, B.L. (1992). Time as a resource and constraint for parents of young children with disabilities: Implications for early intervention services. *Topics in Early Childhood Special Education, 12*(4), 508–527.

Fallon, M., & Harris, M. (1992). Encouraging parent participation in intervention programs. *Transdisciplinary Journal, 2*(2), 141–146.

Gilbert, M., Sciarillo, W., & Von Rembow, D. (1992). Service coordination through case management. In M. Bender & C.A. Baglin (Eds.), *Infants and toddlers: A resource guide for practitioners* (pp. 69–84). San Diego: Singular Publishing Group.

Gilkerson, L., & Young-Holt, C.L. (1992). Supervision and the management of programs serving infants, toddlers, and their families. In E. Fenichel (Ed.), *Learning through supervision and mentorship to support the development of infants and toddlers and their families: A source book* (pp. 113–119). Arlington, VA: National Center for Clinical Infant Programs.

Individuals with Disabilities Education Act (IDEA) of 1990, PL 101-476. (October 30, 1990). Title 20, U.S.C. 1400 et seq: *U.S. Statutes at Large, 104,* 1103–1151.

Ramey, C., Bryant, D., & Suarez, T. (1990). Early intervention: Why, for whom, how, and at what cost? *Clinics in Perinatology, 17*(1), 47–55.

Rosin, P., Whitehead, A., Tuchman, L.I., Jesien, G.S., & Begun, A.L. (1993). *Partnerships in early intervention: A training guide on family-centered care, team building and service coordination.* Madison: Waisman Center, University of Wisconsin–Madison.

Sokoly, M., & Dokecki, P. (1992). Ethical perspectives on family-centered early intervention. *Infants and Young Children, 4*(4), 23–32.

Swan, W.W., & Morgan, J.L. (1993). *Collaborating for comprehensive services for young children and their families: The local interagency coordinating council.* Baltimore: Paul H. Brookes Publishing Co.

Wasik, B.H., Bryant, D.M., & Lyons, C.M. (1990). *Home visiting.* Beverly Hills: Sage Publications.

Whitehead, A., Brown, L., & Rosin, P. (1993). *First glance: Tips for service coordination.* Madison: Wisconsin Personnel Development Project.

Wright, L., & Levac, A.M. (1991). The non-existence of non-compliant families: The influence of Humberto Maturana. *Journal of Advanced Nursing, 17,* 913–917.

Zipper, I.N., Weil, M., & Rounds, K. (1991). *Service coordination for early intervention: Parents and professionals.* Chapel Hill: University of North Carolina at Chapel Hill, Frank Porter Graham Child Development Center.

10

Transitions and Service Coordination

George S. Jesien

◆◆◆

OBJECTIVES

◆◆◆   By completing this chapter, the reader will

- Identify the critical elements of an effective transition process
- Identify the phases of service coordination and the roles that a service coordinator can play in facilitating effective transitions from one program to another
- Identify practices to support parents as they make the transition from one program to another   ◆

All families encounter many transitions throughout their lives. For families of children with disabilities, transitions often take extra planning and can be particularly stressful (Turnbull, Summers, & Brotherson, 1986). The transitions that a family faces during the early years of their child's life often become models for future changes as they move from program to program (Barber, Turnbull, Behr, & Kerns, 1988; Hains, Rosenkoetter, & Fowler, 1991). Early experiences can set the tone for success in future transitions (Rosenkoetter, Hains, & Fowler, 1994), or they can cause a family to dread the repetition, uncertainty, and insecurity of facing the unknown programs or services to come.

Many families have found that periods of transition are especially important but potentially stressful (McDonald, Kysela, Siebert, McDonald, & Chambers, 1989). Support, information, and assistance individualized to individual strengths and needs are critical if a family is to come through these periods successfully (Kilgo, Richard, & Noonan, 1989). A service coordinator can and should serve as a resource, helper, or guide in the transition process. The service coordinator has experience and knowledge that can prove extremely useful to parents as they move from a known program to a new program that may be different in many ways (e.g., types and locations of services, eligibility criteria, schedules, staff-to-consumer or staff-to-child ratio).

Two of the most significant transitions for a family with an infant or a toddler with disabilities are 1) when the child comes home from the hospital, the family adjusts to that child, and the family begins to receive early intervention services from community service providers; and 2) when the child turns 3 years old and he or she begins to receive services from the public school system. Many other transitions can occur as the child and family become involved with follow-up clinics, public or private health care services, private therapists, public or private child care, and, in some instances, mental health and social services providers. The service coordinator can be involved with any and all of these. Timely and appropriate support and information from the service coordinator can facilitate the family's adjustment to future situations and can help them to feel confident about subsequent transitions as well.

Exemplary resources in the area of transition have become available through numerous demonstration and outreach projects funded by a variety of sources, such as the Office of Special Education Programs (OSEP); the National Institute on Disability and Rehabilitation Research (NIDRR); and the Administration for Children, Youth, and Families' Head Start Program. Some of these programs have developed extensive transition models with related resource and training materials. (For information on many of these programs and extensive information on early transitions, the reader is referred to Rosenkoetter et al. [1994], which provides an extensive description of the work of researchers and practitioners in the area of transition as well as lists of projects and other resources, and Neisworth and Fewell [1990], which describes extensive research and provides examples of exemplary practices related to such issues as infants making the transition out of neonatal intensive care units and transition planning for kindergarten and elementary school.)

This chapter concentrates on the role of service coordinators in assisting families with the transitions of their young children with disabilities or special needs. The service coordinator role is still new for many early interventionists. The specific responsibilities related to successful transitions need further study and development.

THE LONS STORY: TRANSITION INTO PRESCHOOL

Shanna Lons has been in a local preschool program for almost 2 months. She entered the program a few months early, before her third birthday, so that she could start with the rest of the class at the beginning of September. Ena, Shanna's mother, has just received a telephone call from her service coordinator from the local birth-to-3 program. The service coordinator telephoned just to check up on how things were going in

Shanna's new program and to ask if there was anything she could do either for Ena or the preschool staff. Shanna had been in a child care program in the mornings previously and was visited on a weekly basis by an early childhood special education teacher from the birth-to-3 program. Ena told the service coordinator how pleased she was with Shanna's adjustments to the full-day program and the new group of children.

She mentioned how the whole transition process had gone so smoothly, beginning with the first meeting with the representative from the local school district and the service coordinator, to her visits to various community programs, and finally to the way Shanna was eased into the daily schedule of the new program. Ena remarked about how the transition plan in the individualized family service plan (IFSP) served as a road map of what to expect, from whom, and when. The plan needed to be changed a few times in order to make allowances for Shanna's early start and a last-minute change in Ena's choice of programs. Ena had decided she preferred the staff and schedule of Shanna's current preschool program over a program upon which they had initially decided.

Ena said that although she had been quite apprehensive about what would happen when her daughter turned 3 years old and they left the birth-to-3 program, she is becoming very comfortable with the staff from the school and preschool. The service coordinator and Ena chatted for a few more minutes before the service coordinator said good-bye, telling Ena that she is available if she needs any help or has any questions. The service coordinator also asked Ena if she would like her to call back in 4 or 5 weeks to check in again. Ena indicated that she would and said good-bye.

TRANSITION AND SERVICE COORDINATION

With variations, this story should be much more common than it is for children and parents making transitions into new programs. Unfortunately, too many parents still know little about what to expect from the next program to which their children will go or about the decisions that they may participate in making (e.g., when and where their children will go to school, which services they will receive). Too many parents feel as though they are being abandoned by people on whom they have grown to trust and depend when they move from a birth-to-3 program to an early childhood program. For many parents, entering the local school system requires that they start over again to figure out a new system and how it operates.

One of the roles of a service coordinator is to help families to have positive transition experiences like Ena's. The primary purpose of this chapter is to explore what service coordinators can do to optimize the chances for successful transitions for children and families.

Part H of IDEA

Part H of the Individuals with Disabilities Education Act (IDEA) makes a number of references to transitions, including the following:

Section 676—Requirements for a statewide system

> Training personnel to coordinate transition services for infants and toddlers with disabilities from an early intervention program under this Part to a preschool program under section 619 of Part B. (8)(D)

Section 677—The IFSP

> The steps to be taken supporting the transition of the toddler with a disability to services provided under Part B of IDEA to the extent such services are considered appropriate. (d)(8)

Section 678—State applications and assurances

> A description of the policies and procedures used to ensure a smooth transition for individuals participating in the early intervention program under this Part who are eligible for participation in preschool programs under Part B, including a description of how the families will be included in the transitional plans and how the lead agency under this Part will notify the appropriate local educational agency or intermediate educational unit in which the child resides and convene, with the approval of the family, a conference between the lead agency, the family, and such agency or unit at least 90 days before the child is eligible for the preschool program under Part B in accordance with state law, and to review the child's program options, for the period commencing on the day a child turns 3 running through the remainder of the school year, and to establish a transition plan. (a)(8)

The law thus recognizes 1) the importance of training to facilitate effective transitions, 2) the need to include a transition plan in the IFSP, and 3) the need for planning procedures and timelines for sharing information among parents and sending and receiving notices about programs. The law also stipulates the need for a meeting during which the principal parties can discuss plans, share pertinent information, and plan next steps.

Additional reference is made in the law to the use of Part H and Part B funds to provide states with flexibility in arranging smooth transitions. Thus, states are allowed to use Part H funding to fund children who turn 3 years old during the school year and conversely to use preschool grant funding to place children who are from 2 to 3 years of age in preschool programs (Part H, Section 679 [3] and Part B, Section 619 [b]). The law also allows the use of an IFSP for children ages 3–5 if it is not prohibited by state law and if local school staff and parents agree (Part B, Section 614 [a][5]). These provisions were placed in the law during the 1991 reauthorization (PL 102-119) to provide states with additional flexibility to help them build more streamlined systems of early intervention for young children with disabilities and their families.

Transition Plan

The transition plan portion of the IFSP is developed by the service coordinator in conjunction with the child's parents. The transition plan describes the steps needed to support the child's transition at age 3 to preschool and/or other appropriate services, as well as any help or information that the family may need. The plan should specify time lines for referral and transfer of pertinent information, with parental consent. It should also address mechanisms and the manner in which the family will be involved in planning for the transition.

Translating these formal requirements of the law into family-friendly procedures and discussions that are individualized for the parent and family is the job of the family's service coordinator. State planning, systems development, and even local interagency agreements can only go so far toward ensuring that the needs of the family are considered. It is up to the service coordinator to adapt and adjust so that the family can exercise their decision-making power and build on their own resources to achieve the best possible transition for themselves and their child.

The parties participating in the transition process typically include the child and family, the sending program or agency, the receiving program or agency, and the service coordinator. The parents' role is pivotal. As the child grows and moves through many programs, surroundings and staff may change, and intervention procedures and materials may vary. The family, however, remains constant. Therefore, it is imperative that the transition process support the parents and that procedures be tailored to meet their needs. Parents should gain useful skills and knowledge during each transition so that they can prepare their child and themselves for transitions later in life when a service coordinator may not be available.

ACTIVITY: *Reverse Chaining*

◆◆◆ Break up into small groups and reread Shanna's story. What must have happened or what events must have taken place to make Ena so positive about Shanna's transition into preschool? Address this question in small groups, then share answers with the group as a whole. ◆

SUCCESSFUL TRANSITIONS

Rosenkoetter et al. (1994) identified some general characteristics of successful transitions. Good transitions are planned and individualized; they involve substantial communication, trust, and shared information; and they empower the parents to advocate for the needs of their child. Thus, although transitions can be times of stress and change, they can also be times of learning and additional support that can pave the way for expanded opportunities for both the child and parents.

Johnson, Chandler, and Kerns (1986) observed that transitions are most effective when they are planned well in advance of actual changes, involve many opportunities for discussions, have parents serving as decision makers, and include plans for both the young child and the family. Kilgo et al. (1989) cautioned that a transition should not be seen as a single event but, rather, as a continuous process that is much more complex than merely transferring records and making placement decisions for a child. Johnson et al. (1986) said that it might be useful to consider the transition process as occurring in three phases: preparation, implementation, and follow-up. Each phase entails specific duties that a service coordinator will need to carry out to optimize the chances for a successful and enabling transition experience for the parents and child.

Preparation

The preparation phase may be the most difficult because it depends so much on the needs, interests, and readiness of the parents to begin thinking about and planning for the next environment that their child is likely to enter. Some parents will want to begin to explore options and learn about the various procedures that will need to be carried out long before an actual transition occurs. Others will be much less interested in the child's next environment and much more focused on what is going on in the present. A research study by Kilgo et al. (1989) indicated that there is an inverse relationship between the severity of a child's disabilities and the parents' readiness to think about the child's future environment. Although the service coordinator will need to interpret each parent's readiness based on the parent's requests and comments, the coordinator must always be sensitive to the parent's concerns. The service coordinator needs to 1) provide opportunities for discussion and for information sharing, and 2) take the lead based on the parent's expressed interests.

In the preparation phase, the service coordinator must have good communication skills and be willing to listen to the parents and their concerns about and hopes for their child. Some parents may have fairly clear ideas about the type of program they are interested in for their child. Others may find the array of options somewhat bewildering. The parents will need support and information that is based on their interests, past knowledge, and motivations to explore additional options.

The service coordinator also must have knowledge about the various program options available in the community; their admission criteria, if any; and any time lines associated with entry. The service coordinator can serve as a bridge between the resources that are available in the community and the referral procedures for gaining access to those resources.

Resources should include formal programs (e.g., early intervention programs) as well as informal resources (e.g., story times, play groups, infant swim classes). It is often the informal resources that provide the broad base of contacts and information that parents need (Dunst, Trivette, & Deal, 1994).

It is also very helpful for the service coordinator to know or to be able to consult with others on the early intervention team in ascertaining the skills that likely will be expected of the child in the next environment. This information will prove useful as the parents begin to anticipate and provide opportunities for the child to learn some of these skills during his or her daily activities. Parents could ask therapists to include activities in their intervention sessions that would facilitate the acquisition of these skills.

In preparing for any transition a child's parents need to be aware of their rights as well as of procedural safeguards to which they are entitled. They also should be aware of the IFSP and individualized education program (IEP) processes, and they should know where they can get additional advocacy assistance in their community or state. Such information may need to be provided in different formats, depending on their preferences and needs.

Finally, the parents should be able to state their perceptions of their child's development and needs. It is hoped that through frequent discussions with their service coordinator, they 1) will have had the opportunity to formulate opinions of their child's strengths and needs, and 2) will feel comfortable expressing their preferences for services and goals for the child. The service coordinator may take on a variety of roles in helping the parents to prepare for any transitions (e.g., information provider, option developer, resource and referral specialist, sounding board). These roles vary over time as the parents' knowledge and concerns change.

ACTIVITY: *Program Differences*

◆ ◆ ◆   Have participants break up into small groups and identify the differences that exist between a birth-to-3 program and an early childhood special education program. Identify differences in environments, expectations of children, and opportunities for parents' input and participation. Discuss how these differences may have an impact on children and families making the transition from one program to the other.   ◆

Implementation

The implementation phase can begin when the first meeting occurs with the family, the sending program staff, and the receiving program staff. It

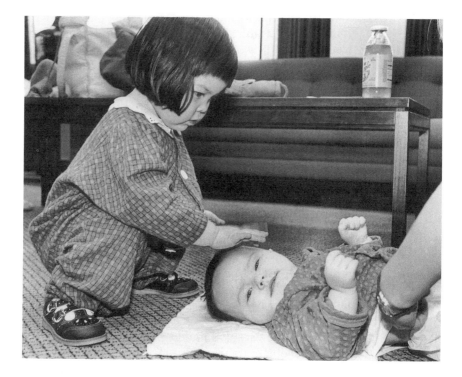

is during this meeting that actual steps will be taken and time lines for the transition will be discussed and decided upon. The service coordinator needs to exercise his or her teaming skills to the extent necessary to ensure that the parents' concerns are heard and addressed. Time lines and respective responsibilities of the sending and receiving programs will need to be determined, and assessment information and information on the strengths and needs of the child will need to be exchanged. Parents may also want to obtain additional information, establish dates to visit programs, or learn of other parents with whom they may talk about possible program options.

Any interagency agreement between a sending program and a receiving program may play an important role in the implementation phase by providing guidelines for when transitions are possible or by determining financial responsibilities for services during periods of transition. It would be best for parents and service coordinators to be aware of any interagency agreements before actual transition activities begin, but this may not always be possible. It is helpful if agreements are written in a way that allows for modifications and adaptations because of the concerns or preferences of a particular child or family. In Shanna's story, Ena changed her mind about the preschool program that her daughter was to attend based on her reactions after visiting the program. It is hoped that transition plans and procedures can be implemented with the flexibility necessary to change as family needs and parent perceptions change.

As the time approaches for the actual transition to occur, the service coordinator can assume another series of roles, depending on the amount of assistance the parents want and need. The service coordinator can be involved minimally if the parents want to assume primary roles in ensuring that 1) the child is ready for the new program or setting, 2) his or her records are transferred, and 3) receiving staff have the benefit of the sending staff's experience with and knowledge of the child. In other instances, the service coordinator may need to play a more active role by helping to schedule meetings and facilitating the transfer of records and information. The important element is to maintain communication so that 1) the child and parents know what to expect, and 2) receiving staff are prepared for their new responsibilities and have the benefit of knowing about the previous program's successes in enhancing the child's development and in addressing the family's needs.

In some instances, the service coordinator will need to serve as a problem solver by helping to mediate between the parents' wishes and the accommodations that can be realistically achieved by the receiving program. Creative solutions may be necessary at times, or new options may need to be developed. Problems may occur, especially when preschool programs for children with disabilities have few options for services in environments with typically developing children. The service coordinator may need to join with parents and other professionals in helping to develop additional community-based options.

Follow-Up

Once the transition has taken place, an important activity for the service coordinator is to follow up with both the family and the receiving program. This contact can serve to reassure the parents that they are still connected with their previous service providers and have not been abandoned. It can be very important to parents who now have to get to know new staff and learn a new system of rules, schedules, and routines. Some parents may use this contact only to exchange stories about recent events and brief comments, whereas others may need time to express their worries, questions, and/or doubts about their child's development or adjustment. Parents also can use this contact as an opportunity to get additional information, review the original transition plan, or merely seek reassurance about how things are going.

Follow-up communications can be very helpful in determining the success of implementation plans as well as of the support services that were put into place for both the child and family. The service coordinator also can follow up with a telephone call to determine which transition procedures and adaptations have been most effective for the family.

This chapter's story of Shanna and Ena depicts a successful transition that was no doubt due in part to the efforts of all participating individuals: the parent, receiving program staff, sending program staff, the service coordinator, and even Shanna because of her efforts to adapt to her new setting.

Parents and service providers hope to make each transition as effective as possible. Some of the expected outcomes, or markers, of effective transitions are listed next. These are offered as a kind of self-test for programs, in the hope that increasing numbers of children and parents will experience effective outcomes with the assistance of early intervention service providers, service coordinators, and other parents.

The following are markers of an effective transition for the child. He or she

- Has developed some knowledge of and/or gained experience in the next environment
- Has developed survival skills that could optimize the potential for rewarding interactions and/or successes in the next environment
- Has a sense of optimism about the next environment

The following are markers of an effective transition for the family. They

- Have a sense that all options were explored in searching for the best possible program, service, or placement for the child
- Feel that they participated fully in the decision-making process with support from the involved service providers
- Received complete, comprehensive, and accurate information about options and about what is best for the child
- Were able to choose among viable options that took the child's needs into account
- Have a sense that a relationship was initiated with a responsive, flexible, and cooperative partner who will work with them in discovering and meeting the child's needs

The following are markers of an effective transition for receiving program staff. They

- Received useful developmental information that will help them to feel confident and able to individualize practices, routines, and materials so the child can enjoy and succeed in the program
- Received information about the family's preferences and concerns regarding the child and the services to be received
- Have a sense that the family feels comfortable with the placement and is looking forward to a positive and beneficial working relationship

These markers may seem like tall orders to achieve during the complex process of transition. Yet, they are attainable if the efforts of all involved parties are directed toward 1) tailoring the transition to the particular needs of the child and family, and 2) establishing and maintaining open lines of communications. The following guidelines are provided to summarize practices of service coordinators that are likely to facilitate effective transitions:

- Provide as much information as possible as soon as parents are interested in finding potential options for their child.
- Encourage parents to visit, observe, and talk with potential future service providers.
- Take cues from the parents about what information they would like and how they would like to get it.
- Develop a transition plan with the parents that maps out steps to be taken, information to be obtained, and people to be responsible for specific tasks.
- Individualize transition procedures based on the family's questions and preferences.
- Establish procedures based on interagency agreements between organizations or agencies with whom the service coordinator works regularly in organizing transitions for children and families.
- Analyze the different demands that potential next environments will place on children; introduce activities that will encourage development of survival skills.
- Provide opportunities for follow up and future support in case the family or the receiving staff have questions after the transition occurs.

SUMMARY

When a child moves from one program or service to another, the transition for the family can be difficult. The service coordinator plays a critical role in facilitating the process for the family. Addressing the needs of the family and defining the responsibilities of the sending and receiving programs and the service coordinator during the phases of preparation, implementation, and follow-up after transitions may be particularly helpful. By attending to the family's need for information, contact, and support, the service coordinator can make the transition process successful for both child and parents and provide the receiving program with the necessary information to work most effectively with the child. Successful outcomes such as those experienced by Ena and her daughter Shanna can be accomplished when providers work closely with parent(s) throughout the transition process.

DISCUSSION QUESTIONS

◆ ◆ ◆   1. What questions or concerns might parents have as their child moves from one program or service provider to another?

2. What are the elements of a responsive and successful transition plan?

3. What kinds of tasks might a service coordinator be called upon to perform in order to obtain positive transition results?   ◆

REFERENCES

Barber, P.A., Turnbull, A.P., Behr, S.K., & Kerns, G.M. (1988). A family systems perspective on early childhood special education. In S.L. Odom & M.B. Karnes (Eds.), *Early intervention for infants and toddlers with handicaps: An empirical base* (pp. 179–198). Baltimore: Paul H. Brookes Publishing Co.

Dunst, C.J., Trivette, C.M., & Deal, A.G. (1994). Resource-based early intervention practices. In C.J. Dunst, C.M. Trivette, & A.G. Deal (Eds.), *Supporting and strengthening families: Vol. 1. Methods, strategies, and practices* (pp. 140–151). Cambridge, MA: Brookline Books

Hains, A.H., Rosenkoetter, S.E., & Fowler, S.A. (1991). Transition planning with families in early intervention programs. *Infants and Young Children, 3,* 38–47.

Individuals with Disabilities Education Act (IDEA) of 1990, PL 101-476. (October 30, 1990). Title 20, U.S.C. 1400 et seq: *U.S. Statutes at Large, 104,* 1103–1151.

Individuals with Disabilities Education Act Amendments of 1991, PL 102-119. (October 7, 1991). Title 20, U.S.C. 1400 et seq: *U.S. Statutes at Large, 105,* 587–608.

Johnson, T.E., Chandler, L.K., & Kerns, G.M. (1986). What are parents saying about family involvements in school transitions? A retrospective transition interview. *Journal of the Division for Early Childhood, 11,* 10–17.

Kilgo, J.L., Richard, N., & Noonan, M.J. (1989). Teaming for the future: Integrating transition planning with early intervention services for young children with special needs and their families. *Infants and Young Children, 2*(2), 37–48.

McDonald, L., Kysela, G.M., Siebert, P., McDonald, S., & Chambers, J. (1989). Parent perspectives: Transition to preschool. *Teaching Exceptional Children, 22,* 4–8.

Neisworth, J.T., & Fewell, R.R. (Eds.). (1990). Transition [Special issue]. *Topics in Early Childhood Special Education, 2*(4).

Rosenkoetter, S.E., Hains, A.H., & Fowler, S.A. (1994). *Bridging early services for children with special needs and their families: A practical guide for transition planning.* Baltimore: Paul H. Brookes Publishing Co.

Turnbull, A.P., Summers, J.A., & Brotherson, M.J. (1986). Family life cycle: Theoretical and empirical implications and future directions for families with mentally retarded members. In J.J. Gallagher & P.M. Vietze (Eds.), *Families of handicapped persons: Research, programs, and policy issues* (pp. 45–65). Baltimore: Paul H. Brookes Publishing Co.

11

FUTURE CHALLENGES IN EARLY INTERVENTION

George S. Jesien

OBJECTIVES

◆ ◆ ◆   By completing this chapter the reader will

- Have an awareness of the historical development of the early intervention field
- Understand the importance of parent–professional partnerships and interagency collaboration in shaping the present status of early intervention policy and practice
- Be able to identify a series of challenges that the early intervention field faces ◆

Since the early intervention field first began to develop in the early 1960s, it has experienced meteoric growth in numerous interrelated areas, including parent advocacy, research, policy development, and recommended practices. Increasing federal and state governmental investment in programs for children with disabilities has played a key role in spurring this growth, both in research and services for young children with special needs and their families (Smith & McKenna, 1994). The field has served as a social experiment in developing effective strategies for providing resources to a significant segment of society.

The development of interventions and program strategies can be traced to 1968, to the beginnings of the Handicapped Children's Early Education Program (HCEEP), enacted by the Handicapped Children's Early Education Act, PL 90-538 (Hebbler, Smith, & Black, 1991). The concepts on which the HCEEP program was built included addressing the overall development of the child, parent participation, community-based programs, and interdisciplinary services. These principles have shaped the continuing development of research and practice over the past 3 decades and have set the stage for the field's continuing progress. More recently, concepts such as parent–professional partnership, service coordination, and interagency collaboration have become part of the inventory of critical elements of high-quality services. This list serves as a template for the provision of comprehensive and coordinated services for young children with disabilities and their families. As the new concepts are applied in the practice of early intervention, the field will face a series of challenges that will guide its future development.

ONE COMMUNITY'S RESPONSE—REPLICATED MANY TIMES OVER

The meeting was to be called to order at 2 P.M. The 15 members of the Anywhere County Interagency Coordinating Council were ready to begin their third year as the county's coordinating body and advisory group for young children with special needs and their families. The council's charge is to provide a forum for discussing and analyzing interagency practices and county policy regarding children birth through age 6 who may have special needs and their families. The council has decided that addressing the needs of any group of children whose optimal development is challenged or threatened is appropriate for discussion during council meetings. Their role is purely advisory, but because members—both agency heads and parents—have invested their time and effort, the council has been very influential in the county.

The council originally comprised 12 members, but 3 additional members were added 18 months ago to provide better representation for the diverse cultural and racial groups in the community, including African American, Latino, and Hmong. The three members were added because of their standing with their respective communities and their work in community-based outreach efforts. The rest of the council is composed of three parents who have or have had children in the early intervention system, the heads of a number of agencies in the county including the county executive, a local elected council person, a pediatrician who also works in the neonatal intensive care unit in the county, the director of the local United Cerebral Palsy Association, a school district official, a Head Start director, a public health official, the director of the local child care resource and referral agency, and a representative from a local 2-year vocational school that trains child development associates and also has a program for occupational therapy associates. Although some of the members knew each other before joining the council, the council represents a unique opportunity for county officials to regularly meet to focus on the needs of very young children and their families.

The council has had its ups and downs over the last 3 years. Disagreements have arisen, for example, over whether the county should charge a sliding fee schedule for services; whether parents should serve as service coordinators; the most effective strategies for helping children make the transition from birth-to-3 programs to Head Start, to the school system, and to other nursery schools and child care providers; and the degree of inclusiveness in county child care centers. For each issue, however, the council has reached a resolution that is at least acceptable to, if not enthusiastically embraced by, all members.

After each resolution, the council has grown in stature in the community, and members have felt more confident dealing with subsequent issues. Members have also begun to place more trust in each other. As individual members have been willing to bend and see the other sides of issues, the more they have realized that the council was in fact working for the betterment of all children in the county and that each agency had to understand its role in the effectiveness of the overall system.

One method that the council has found instructive for analyzing issues and generating possible solutions has been to look at situations from the perspectives of families—the consumers of services. For instance, when the council anticipated restructuring its identification practices, it had to face several difficult issues. The Public Health Agency had its own process; the schools had another for identifying children with disabilities; Head Start had a third system; and the newly developing birth-to-3 system had yet another. Each used different forms, asked similar but different questions of parents, and had difficulties identifying children in varying cultural groups in the county. In the process of revamping its identification process, the council had to deal with turf issues of the respective agencies, the inertia of established practice, and the reluctance of some agencies to compromise. However, by approaching this issue from the perspective of a family seeking information and assistance for their child, the council came to recognize how fragmented its system was and the importance of identifying ways to simplify the process. The solution was not found in the first meeting; however, with time the county ultimately established a single point of entry for all families who requested help for their children.

Parent input on the Child-Find and identification process was invaluable. Parent comments and experiences provided new information and served as a catalyst encouraging other council members to look for more effective ways to identify children. The presence of parents also enhanced cooperation because parents had less interest in established or organizational boundaries and were more directly focused on what they perceived as most beneficial for their children. The development of a single point of entry provided the council with another successful resolution that had a positive impact on all services in the county and heightened members' resolve to face future issues.

The next issue that came before the council was of that of determining a model of service coordination. At that time, there was no uniformity to the service modes in use: in some instances, a dedicated service coordinator carried out the responsibilities; in others, a primary service provider filled that role; and in still others, a program hired parents to serve as service coordinators. Some of the service coordinators were county employees, whereas others were employed by provider agencies. There were numerous advantages and disadvantages associated with each manner of service coordination.

The question before the council at the 2 P.M. meeting was whether to move toward countywide standardizing of service coordination or to keep the options then current. The council members had already assigned a task force to analyze the issue, had asked for input from state officials, and had gathered information from federally funded projects that dealt with service coordination. The council was to receive a report from the task force at the meeting and also hear from providers and parents who had opinions on the issue. As council members prepared for the meeting, no one knew what the final recommendation to the county would be, but they felt assured of obtaining the information they needed, and that the outcome would be based on an open and thorough discussion and would reflect, in great part, the best interests of the county's families.

ROLE OF PL 99-457 AND PART H OF THE INDIVIDUALS WITH DISABILITIES EDUCATION ACT (IDEA), PL 101-476

The continuing development of the early intervention field since the 1960s attests to its breadth, vitality, and richness both in conceptual growth and in its ability to respond to emerging needs. The passage of the Education of the Handicapped Act Amendments of 1986 (PL 99-457), including the original Part H program, represented a culmination of research results, recommended practice, and experiences gained from numerous models, demonstrations, and research efforts across the United States (J.J. Gallagher, Trohanis, & Clifford, 1989). A wide array of participants, including parents, early intervention providers, researchers, and administrators, contributed to the law's creation. The law also provided an opportunity for officials from the health, education, and social services sectors to focus on the challenges faced by families who had infants and toddlers with disabilities or who were at risk of developmental delay.

PL 99-457 encased the prevailing elements of recommended practice into legislated policy that provided incentives for states to develop comprehensive, statewide systems of service and support for the just-mentioned segments of the population. The 14 components of the statewide system identified in the law outlined an all-encompassing approach to services that includes the participation of individuals from the social services, health, and education sectors—sectors whose services are crucial to the well-being and support of families and children with special needs. The law also provided for a melding of resources from federal, state, and local sources, along with services from the private sector to bring these resources to bear on the challenges facing families in rearing young children with special needs (Smith & Strain, 1988).

Early intervention has moved dramatically and systematically from individual experimental models to efforts to validate and replicate these models and to broader national attempts at investigating statewide variations and adaptations. In the process, the field has matured, predicated on a set of commonly accepted principles, recommended practices, and a commitment to flexibility based on local need. If early intervention continues to succeed on a broad basis, it may well serve as a model for support and service systems for children and families of older children and families facing a range of challenges including poverty, substance abuse, child abuse and neglect, and other crises.

The pieces are now in place. Policy has been tested, refined, and developed, backed by a growing body of research supporting the directions the field is taking. Funding sources have been identified, and a significant segment of the public is convinced that resources *do* need to be allocated on local, state, and national levels to support families and children's development. The public is also becoming increasingly aware of the critical importance of meeting the needs of infants with special needs during their foundational years.

PL 99-457 and its reauthorization—the Individuals with Disabilities Education Act of 1990 (PL 101-476)—changed the face of agency interactions and the structure of the very conversations that agencies and their staffs have with each other. Whereas once agencies worked independently, Part H of IDEA has brought about an unprecedented need for agencies to plan together and to coordinate their efforts with the efforts of others in the fields of early intervention and child development (Swan & Morgan, 1993). These new interactions will likely lead to profound changes in the way providers work with each other and the families they serve. We may truly be seeing the beginning of an early intervention community linked by a common interest in providing appropriate services to young children with special needs and their families. This community is built on the notion of interdependence within the system (R.J. Gallagher, LaMontagne, & Johnson, 1994).

PL 99-457 has permanently installed two additional concepts in the practice of early intervention: parent–professional partnership and interagency collaboration, both evolving out of past experiences with successful early intervention programs. These concepts have guided and will continue to guide the expansion of early intervention practice and the next wave of national, state, and local development. These concepts are discussed further in the sections following.

PARENT–PROFESSIONAL PARTNERSHIP

The hallmark of PL 99-457 has been the hoped-for partnership with parents of children with special needs at all levels of early intervention, from public policy development at national, state, and local levels to team participation in planning and designing specific early intervention services for a particular family. Parents have also helped to design, coordinate, and staff other components required by the law. Parents have become active in developing information resources; participating on committees and task forces that establish state guidelines; designing public awareness campaigns; and designing and implementing personnel preparation activities. Parents have assumed a much more equitable partnership role with professionals in designing and developing the present early intervention field than in any other modern social program.

Indeed, the early intervention field has redefined the traditional roles of providers, professionals, and experts as they relate to families and consumers (Buysse & Wesley, 1993). These new roles acknowledge the key part the consumer plays in the success or failure of any intervention—the reciprocal need of one for the other. Because services and supports to families are in part based on the relationship that is established, maintained, and nourished between providers and parents, services need to be conceptualized to facilitate relationship building (Kalmanson & Seligman, 1992). Services need to be structured to allow for mutual esteem and learning to evolve over time as both parties resolve problems, learn from each other, and grow to respect their respective strengths, knowledge, and concerns for the future. Such a relationship requires frequent, regular, and long-term involvement. Early intervention, as currently conceptualized and practiced, supports the development of relationships between providers and parents for the time that the child receives services, and provides for the transition of parent connectedness to subsequent providers (Rosenkoetter, Hains, & Fowler, 1994).

Although tremendous variability exists in the character of parent participation across the United States, the widespread goal of fuller participation by parents in the early intervention process permeates much of the field. As this social effort continues in years to come, the results bear watching. Resources for training, research, model development, and demonstrations have been dedicated to studying and developing recommended practices that reflect parents' expanding participation.

As parents continue to grow into their new roles on policy boards, as participants in preservice and in-service training, and as hired staff members who provide intake or service coordination for families, the emerging systems will increasingly take into account the desires and recommendation of parents. What effect will this have on the future development of the system as it is pushed to be ever more responsive to families? What will be the next phases of parent participation? How will this structure affect the field's development and evolution? In what other ways can parents be involved? As program coordinators? Ombudspersons for programs? Elected policy makers? Researchers? Or state-level officials? These and similar questions will be resolved in future years as parent participation becomes more established.

A related question involves how parents who have participated in early intervention programs will affect the special education programs into which many of their children will move. How will the partnership established in early intervention shape and mold the interactions between parents and school systems in the future? Will school systems be prepared to deal with parents who are accustomed to being consulted and playing a proactive—and in many instances, a guiding—role as members of decision-making teams who establish collaborative partnerships to plan and execute the program over time?

Full parent participation in the Anywhere County Interagency Coordinating Council, described at the beginning of this chapter, clearly influenced the council's decision-making process, as well as the strategies used to address issues. Continuing and growing parent participation based on an equitable partnership with professionals will serve as a major resource in the future development of early intervention policy and practice. The changing needs of children and families will keep the field dynamic and will help to ensure that policy and practice remain flexible and responsive to these changes (R.J. Gallagher, LaMontagne, et al., 1994).

ACTIVITY: *Parental Roles*

◆ ◆ ◆

Have participants make two lists. The first list should comprise all the roles that they know of that parents of children with special needs have assumed in early intervention programs at the local community or state levels. The second list should comprise all the other roles that they think parents might play in the future as the early intervention field continues to develop. Ask questions such as the following to stimulate discussion:

1. What would it take for the roles in the second list to become a reality or more widely accepted?
2. What obstacles make it difficult for parents to play the roles on the second list?
3. What supports will parents need to take on additional roles if they choose?
4. How will professionals or providers need to change to support parents taking on additional roles?
5. Are there roles parents should not take? Can early intervention policies go too far in encouraging parent–professional partnerships? ◆

INTERAGENCY COLLABORATION

The future for early intervention is challenged by the continuing trend toward and need for increasing collaboration among policy, state planning, and service provider agencies. Agencies will need well-developed mechanisms to work with other agencies, collaborative service plans, and methods for cofunding or mingling their financial and human resources to provide the necessary services and supports. Efforts such as the early intervention program under Part H of IDEA; the Child and Adolescent Systems Service Program (CASSP), approved in the mid-1980s as a federal set-aside in states' mental health funds; the Family Preservation and Support Act (PL 103-66) passed by Congress in 1993; Head Start; and the Community Integrated Service System (CISS) established by the Maternal and Child Health Bureau, all require closer collaboration and interagency functioning than in the past.

As organizations from the health, education, and social services sectors continue to converge and work together on problems facing children and families, a realignment or restructuring of the organizations themselves may emerge. Family and child issues cut across the three sectors. The duplication and fragmentation that occur now are major sources of frustration to parents and may be partly to blame for the failures parents sometimes experience in confronting the current service structure. The closer working relationships fostered by the search for more effective ways to serve families could conceivably lead to multiple services provided by one agency that cut across health, education, and social services needs. We may be witnessing the emergence of new structures or a new blend of organizations that addresses problems on a more holistic basis and reforms local, state, and national service and administrative structures.

Early intervention can serve at the forefront of this development. Addressing the needs of young children and families by necessity requires a more noncategorical approach and demands flexibility and attention to a broad range of needs. As agencies review their procedures and ability to respond to their consumers, areas of overlap may need to be reviewed and new structures developed that cross the traditional service boundaries (e.g., health clinics are now increasingly placed in school buildings). Early intervention blends social services and developmental supports and health and medical services. The challenge will be to keep focused on the need for easily accessible, coordinated, and comprehensive services, as well as straightforward systems that families can understand.

The presence of agency heads and providers on the Anywhere County Council clearly helped the council to see issues more comprehensively, in addition to generating more novel solutions to problems than might have been possible from a narrower spectrum of the community.

Interagency collaboration does not guarantee solutions, but it helps ensure more comprehensive approaches to problem solving as well as a broader participation in that process than in the past.

UPCOMING CHALLENGES

Now that resources and a system for national implementation of early intervention have been put in place, a new set of challenges surfaces. Demographic and economic changes and an emerging new morbidity pose serious new difficulties for the field. As problems such as poverty, drug use, and domestic violence in the United States deepen and as technological advances increase the survivability of low birth weight infants, some with residual physical challenges or developmental delays (Baumeister, Kupsta, & Klindworth, 1990), many families are increasingly vulnerable and in need of comprehensive services and support. The following section of this chapter outlines some of the challenges the field must confront.

Continuing Flexibility

Flexibility, responsiveness, and a willingness to experiment have been major characteristics of the early intervention field. The field's ongoing success can be attributed to its pursuit of recommended practice, its willingness to cross traditional professional boundaries in health and education, and its ability to enact innovative statewide and national policy. One of the field's major advantages has been its relative youth. In this regard, the tendency of early intervention to remain flexible has been due not only to its focus on the family but also to the absence of longstanding, crystallized, and formal bureaucratic structures. The bureaucracies dedicated to early intervention have only recently emerged. As the field and services mature and state and local systems are established, the challenge will be to ensure that rigid bureaucracies do not emerge that limit flexibility and responsiveness. The danger is that burdensome rules and regulations will replace local responsiveness to the unique needs of families. For example, there is a fear that one-size-fits-all answers may develop. One question that surfaces frequently at the local level concerns defining what constitutes sufficient or base-level services. The answer often given now is that it depends on the needs of the child and family. Yet, many would like to see standards set for frequency and intensity of services. Such a standard, if set as a minimum, could quickly become the maximum and any deviation from it would need to be justified.

Maintaining the flexibility to respond creatively to the individual needs of families is an ongoing challenge for early intervention programs. Remaining responsive will partly depend on the willingness of local and state officials to continually seek out ways to improve services and make them more supportive. As J.J. Gallagher, Harbin, Eckland, and

Clifford (1994) have stated, the intent of PL 99-457 has been to provide substantial flexibility or "freedom within structure" (p. 240). The challenge for the field will be to maintain sufficient freedom to remain flexible and responsive as the structure grows.

Defining a Professional

Another challenge for the field is the evolving definition of the professional in early intervention. There is a simultaneous need in early intervention for highly specialized personnel in the various areas of development, such as communication and motor and cognitive development, and well-trained generalists who understand overall child development and the role of the family. Both types of professionals are in short supply. Many families with infants with multiple needs have a plethora of professionals in their lives, which may inadvertently increase stress in the family by the need to contend with and coordinate multiple interventions and schedule numerous appointments. The close linkage among developmental areas in the life of an infant underscores the need for professionals who can provide holistic, integrated services that take into account the manifold and blended needs of infants and their families. Interdisciplinary training is one way to help ensure that professionals understand multiple areas of development and the roles and functions of professionals in allied fields.

Another alternative is to develop a new profile of the early interventionist as a professional who has a range of training in communication and motor and cognitive development, as well as a solid understanding of the health needs of the young child and the role of family members in the child's development. Such a professional could truly be considered an early interventionist who brings a wide scope of pediatric knowledge to the family. Clearly, this type of person would not have the more specialized knowledge of professionals in their respective fields and would therefore need to be supported by such professionals.

Training programs will need to bring expertise and faculty from multiple departments, along with the knowledge base appropriate to the development of young children and families (Featherman, 1993). However, changing the departmental structure of universities can be a long and difficult process. In the meantime, the amount and extent of interdisciplinary training will need to increase across the United States to provide the necessary skills and knowledge to the next cohort of professionals working with families.

Recognizing Diversity

The cultural diversity of the U.S. population is increasing, with early intervention service providers assisting more and more families from varied ethnic backgrounds (Lynch & Hanson, 1992). How can the field respond to the added demands and complexity of this diversity? The effect of any response will be mitigated unless the diversity of personnel in the field also increases. At present the system is out of balance, with few people from racially and culturally diverse backgrounds providing services to populations with ever-increasing diversity (Lynch & Hanson, 1993). The challenge is to attract, train, and place people of diverse backgrounds throughout the system, from direct services provider to state and national leadership positions. Those interested in young children will need career ladders supporting progress through the requisite education to obtain the credentials to serve as professionals in the field. Multilevel strategies will need to be developed to increase the public's awareness of professional fields associated with early intervention. These may need to be directed at high schools where students make many decisions that can affect their potential entry into college programs. For example, deciding not to take the prerequisite science or mathematics courses in high school may, in effect, close out the possibilities of becoming a physical therapist later in college.

Another more-immediate strategy that may be effective while awaiting results from longer-term efforts is to use community individuals from the respective cultural and racial backgrounds in early intervention programs as liaison individuals. Programs can provide these individuals training in early intervention and then have them serve as bridges to the communities. In this way the cultural values of the respective group can be represented to the service providers and the trained individuals can provide outreach to the community by translating and adapting intervention strategies. Parents who have or had children in the program may also serve as bridge builders to diverse communities.

Increasing Services to Those at Risk

Part H of IDEA was initially worded so that states had the option of including children at risk in the definition of children eligible for early intervention services in their state. The definition was also left up to state discretion. Thus far, only a handful of states include children at risk. Clearly many children other than those with developmental delays or conditions that are likely to lead to developmental delay need comprehensive, family-centered services. The need for family supports and services for families that are challenged because of poverty, health risks, substance abuse, or violence is also obvious. The central question is how to provide needed broad-based and effective services within the context of obtainable resources. Resources will need to combine funds from local, state, and national entities. Part H provides a number of options for expanding services to children at risk and their families.

Alternatively, Part H itself could be restructured to further encourage states to include children at risk. States could be required to serve children at risk, or financial incentives could be increased for states to include such children in their eligibility definition. Increasing the requirements on states, however, would be contrary to the tradition of Part H, which has been to provide states considerable discretion. The removal of a perceived obstacle may also serve as an incentive. Allowing states flexibility to decide which services children at risk would receive or allowing them to serve a portion of the children at risk may serve as incentives. Rather than entitling all children at risk to all services, the law might allow states to select some base service such as service coordination for all children, with the remaining services to be provided according to available resources rather than on an entitlement basis. Some precedent exists in that many programs for populations at risk operate on a to-the-degree possible standard, rather than an entitlement approach. However, many in the field would be reluctant to step back from the present entitlement to services provided under Part H. Others would be concerned that without the infusion of considerable new resources, the quality of services to already-eligible children would suffer if there were significant increases in the number of children to be served.

Another option is to further develop collaborative efforts with other agencies that have an impact on the health and well-being of young children and families to create a web of services that supports families. These other agencies such as Head Start, the Maternal and Child Health Bureau, welfare, and Social Security could work to develop collaborative procedures that would assist families and children at risk to receive the services they need in the most effective way. Furthermore, interagency mechanisms need to be established so that families receive the necessary resources and support. The search for effective ways to extend the benefits of early intervention to the widening population of those needing services will be a continuing challenge for early intervention professionals, parents, and law makers in the coming years.

Blending Formal and Informal Supports

An emerging challenge for the early intervention field is that of maintaining and further developing a blend of formal and informal support systems for families. Often as assistance has been formalized, rich and varied informal supports have been pushed aside and replaced. Assistance to families is more likely to be beneficial if it promotes families' ability to use existing resources and support networks to meet their needs (Raab, Davis, & Trepanier, 1993). Recent studies (Dunst, Trivette, & Deal, 1994; Dunst, Trivette, Starnes, Hamby, & Gordon, 1993) show the importance and effectiveness of informal supports for families. Such supports grant parents more of a feeling of control over the services they receive and the development of their children. There is a continuing need in early intervention to develop and nurture a blend of informal family and community resources and supports with more formalized and

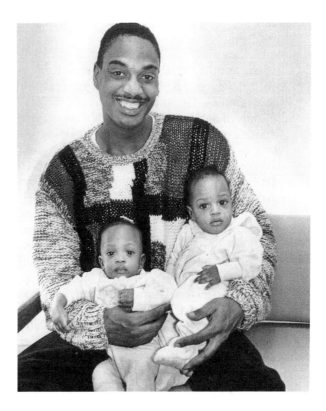

necessary intervention services. The critical factor in guiding this will be the needs and desires of the individual family as well as the resources available to them within their extended family, from friends, and from the community.

Meeting the Need for Additional Resources

Services are still not available for all those children and families who are eligible for them or need them. Although early intervention has received increasing financial federal and state supports over the years, universal coverage is still a goal to be reached. As the U.S. population ages, it may become more difficult to garner the necessary resources to provide for the development of very young children. There is a risk that increased competition from the needs of an aging population may make resources for early intervention more scarce. A wide-based advocacy community will need to ensure that legislators and the public are kept aware of the critical needs for developmental services for young children with disabilities and supports for their families. Research needs to build on past findings to firmly establish the cost-effectiveness and long-term benefits of early intervention.

Resolving Disputes

As the law and regulations concerning early intervention become established, another challenge for the system will be to avoid becoming overly litigious. The law entitles services and supports to children and their families. Questions concerning degree, intensity, frequency, and location of services and supports will inevitably arise. The hope is that when disputes arise, responses can be developed in which both parties work to develop mutually agreeable solutions that provide for the optimal development of the child within the financial resources available. If parties reach an impasse, impartial mediation by a knowledgeable third party can, in most cases, bring the sides together to a workable solution. Decision making is premised on individual solutions that address the concerns and priorities of the family and yet build on the family's existing resources. Use of informal supports is also likely to lessen the demand for only formalized professional services. According to Dunst, Trivette, and Deal (1994), these informal supports can be as effective, if not more effective, than the formal professional services that are in such short supply.

Education in general and special education specifically have become much more litigious over the years. Too often parents and schools have found themselves in adversarial roles that can make it more difficult for the system to be responsive. The partnership paradigm established as a foundation for early intervention may help the field avoid dependence upon the courts to define the details of responsibility. Many states are now developing mediational systems to resolve disputes (Place, 1994). The critical factor in local and state disputes will be to build and maintain trust among the parties involved that the best is being sought for the child and family and that all parties are struggling ultimately to meet the needs of families with the combined resources of local providers, families, and the local community. Clearly, procedural safeguards will need to remain in place. But, one hopes that they will serve as the tool of last resort, rather than the first line of action when conflicts develop.

Expanding the Interchange of Information

The development of early intervention in the United States is rich in lessons and information that could be usefully shared with other countries. Information on the role of parents, interdisciplinary teamwork, training programs, and policy development procedures could assist other countries embarking on programs to serve, or continue to serve, very young children and their families. Similarly, other countries' experiences in developing support systems could provide policy makers and service providers potentially interesting elements that could be incorporated into U.S. systems. Investigation of examples from both developed and developing countries could enrich the discussion of ways to enhance the present system in the United States and continue to improve early intervention's responsiveness to diverse needs. As the U.S. population continues to grow more diverse, a deeper understanding of other systems and their components is sure to increase understanding of the needs and expectations of families from diverse cultural backgrounds.

The interchange between American providers and parents and those from other countries can not only enrich our respective systems but increase the dialogue over how we address the needs of young children and families on a global level. The advocacy and example of countries devoting time and energy to the youngest of their populations can serve as a powerful motivator to countries who have not yet seen this population as a priority. Attention to infants and toddlers with disabilities may also help garner attention for older children and adults with disabilities. Increasing the contact and dialogue among early interventionists worldwide is certain to be of mutual help and assistance in seeking the most effective means possible to serve people with disabilities.

ACTIVITY: *Developing an Intervention Program*

◆ ◆ ◆

Given the list of challenges presented in this chapter, develop a description of a local early intervention program for the year 2000. Provide a list of elements or components that should comprise the program and a list of characteristics describing it. Questions you may want to ask yourself to help guide your program are the following:

1. How do families enter into the program? What are their initial experiences?
2. What is the program's staffing pattern? What education, training, and work experience do staff members possess?
3. What relationships does the program have with other community agencies?
4. What are the program's advisory and administrative structures?
5. What roles do parents play in the program? ◆

SUMMARY

Part H of IDEA has served as an instrument of reform, reinvention, and evolutionary progress for professional practice and the structure of early intervention (J.J. Gallagher, Harbin, et al., 1994). The law has also served as a vehicle for providing additional resources, not only to deliver services but also to build organizational infrastructure for new collaborative relationships at the family, community, state, and national levels. The new knowledge and practices developed within early intervention, many of which have been discussed in this book, pose exciting and ambitious developments and opportunities for parents, service providers, and others interested in early intervention to review and study. If early intervention continues to address challenges in years to come with equal energy and sensitivity, the field will serve as a major source of ideas, practices, and policies for many other sectors of society. As gratifying as the progress since the 1960s has been, the years surrounding the turn of the century offer even more potential for positively influencing broad sectors of the U.S. population and directly affecting the health and well-being of the nation.

We in early intervention live and work in a period filled with challenges and also tremendous promise to effect positive change and ensure the well-being of major segments of the population. We have set a framework of cooperation and open dialogue of which we can be proud. This tradition of partnership should serve us all well into the 21st century.

DISCUSSION QUESTIONS

1. What other challenges (in addition to those mentioned in the chapter) now exist or are likely to develop in the coming years that early intervention will need to address?
2. Pick any one of the challenges described in the text and discuss the likely outcomes if positive solutions are not found. Examples: If greater diversity among service providers is not achieved. . . . If financial and human resources do not increase but in fact decrease. . . .
3. Which of the challenges discussed in the text do you see as the highest priority and why? What actions on local, state, or national levels should be taken to address it? ◆

REFERENCES

Baumeister, A.A., Kupsta, F., & Klindworth, L.M. (1990). New morbidity: Implications for prevention of children's disabilities. *Exceptionality, 1*(1), 1–16.

Buysse, V., & Wesley, P.W. (1993). The identity crisis in early childhood special education: A call for professional role clarification. *Topics in Early Childhood Special Education, 3*(4), 418–429.

Dunst, C.J., Trivette, C.M., & Deal, A.G. (1994). Enabling and empowering families. In C.J. Dunst, C.M. Trivette, & A.G. Deal (Eds.), *Supporting and strengthening families: Vol. 1. Methods, strategies and practices* (pp. 2–11). Cambridge, MA: Brookline Books.

Dunst, C.J., Trivette, C.M., Starnes, A.L., Hamby, D.W., & Gordon, N.J. (1993). *Building and evaluating family support initiatives: A national study of programs for persons with developmental disabilities.* Baltimore: Paul H. Brookes Publishing Co.

Education of the Handicapped Act Amendments of 1986, PL 99-457. (October 8, 1986). Title 20, U.S.C. 1400 et seq: *U.S. Statutes at Large, 100,* 1145–1177.

Featherman, D.L. (1993). What does society need from higher education? In *An American imperative: Higher expectations for higher education*. A Report of the Wingspread Group on Higher Education. Racine, WI: The Johnson Foundation.

Gallagher, J.J., Harbin, G., Eckland, J., & Clifford, R. (1994). State diversity and policy implementation: Infants and toddlers. In L.J. Johnson, R.J. Gallagher, M.J. LaMontagne, & J.B. Jordan, J.J. Gallagher, P.L. Hutinger, & M.B. Karnes (Eds.), *Meeting early intervention challenges: Issues from birth to three* (2nd ed., pp. 235–250). Baltimore: Paul H. Brookes Publishing Co.

Gallagher, J.J., Trohanis, P.L., & Clifford, R.M. (Eds.). (1989). *Policy implementation and PL 99-457: Planning for young children with special needs*. Baltimore: Paul H. Brookes Publishing Co.

Gallagher, R.J., LaMontagne, M.J., & Johnson, L.J. (1994). Early intervention: The collaborative challenge. In L.J. Johnson, R.J. Gallagher, M.J. LaMontagne, & J.B. Jordan, J.J. Gallagher, P.L. Hutinger, & M.B. Karnes (Eds.), *Meeting early intervention challenges: Issues from birth to three* (2nd ed., pp. 279–287). Baltimore: Paul H. Brookes Publishing Co.

Handicapped Children's Early Education Act, PL 90-538. (September 30, 1968). Title 20, U.S.C. 621 et seq: *U.S. Statutes at Large, 82,* 901–902.

Hebbler, K.M., Smith, B.J., & Black, T.L. (1991). Federal early childhood special education policy: A model for the improvement of services for children with disabilities. *Exceptional Children, 58*(2), 104–112.

Individuals with Disabilities Education Act (IDEA) of 1990, PL 101-476. (October 30, 1990). Title 20, U.S.C. 1400 et seq: *U.S. Statutes at Large, 104,* 1103–1151.

Kalmanson, B., & Seligman, S. (1992). Family–provider relationships: The basis of all interventions. *Infants and Young Children, 4*(4), 46–52.

Lynch, E.W., & Hanson, M.J. (Eds.). (1992). *Developing cross-cultural competence: A guide to working with young children and their families*. Baltimore: Paul H. Brookes Publishing Co.

Lynch, E.W., & Hanson, M.J. (1993). Changing demographics: Implications for training in early intervention. *Infants and Young Children, 6*(1), 50–55.

Place, P.A. (1994). Social policy and family autonomy. In L.J. Johnson, R.J. Gallagher, M.J. LaMontagne, & J.B. Jordan, J.J. Gallagher, P.L. Hutinger, & M.B. Karnes (Eds.), *Meeting early intervention challenges: Issues from birth to three* (2nd ed., pp. 265–278). Baltimore: Paul H. Brookes Publishing Co.

Raab, M.L., Davis, M.S., & Trepanier, A.M. (1993). Resources versus services: Changing the focus of intervention for infants and young children. *Infants and Young Children, 5*(3), 1–11.

Rosenkoetter, S.E., Hains, A.H., & Fowler, S.A. (1994). *Bridging early services for children with special needs and their families: A practical guide for transition planning*. Baltimore: Paul H. Brookes Publishing Co.

Smith, B.J., & McKenna, P. (1994). Early intervention public policy: Past, present, and future. In L.J. Johnson, R.J. Gallagher, M.J. LaMontagne, & J.B. Jordan, J.J. Gallagher, P.L. Hutinger, & M.B. Karnes (Eds.), *Meeting early intervention challenges: Issues from birth to three* (2nd ed., pp. 251–264). Baltimore: Paul H. Brookes Publishing Co.

Smith, B.J., & Strain, P.S. (1988). Early childhood special education in the next decade: Implementing and expanding PL 99-457. *Topics in Early Childhood Special Education, 8*(1), 37–47.

Swan, W.W., & Morgan, J.L. (1993). *Collaborating for comprehensive services for young children and their families: The local interagency coordinating council*. Baltimore: Paul H. Brookes Publishing Co.

INDEX

◆◆◆